THE
ALMANAC OF
BACK PAIN
TREATMENTS

D1555711

Julie Zimmerman, PT

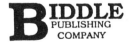

BIDDLE
PUBLISHING
COMPANY

PO Box 1305 #103, Brunswick, Maine 04011

Copyright © 1991

by

Biddle Publishing Company

Publisher's Cataloging in Publication Data

1 - Zimmerman, Julie

2 - The Almanac of Back Pain Treatments

3 - Bibliography, Appendix B

   Includes Index

4 - Alternative treatment of back pain

   Backache

   Diagnosis of back pain

   Health, back care

   Holistic treatment of back pain

   Medical self - care

   Medical treatment of back pain

   Self - care, health

   Treatment of back pain

Library of Congress Catalog Card Number 90 - 85650

ISBN 1 - 879418 - 03 - 7

Dedication

To Susan, Lloyd and all the other health professionals who join their chronic pain patients in the search for answers

and

To Sandy, Barbara and all the other friends and family members who respect the decision to end the search

Back Pain

Lumbar spasm.
Clenching of teeth around the spine.
It can come on suddenly, with
Devastating clarity, not easily confused
With other pronunciations.

Everything grinds to a halt.
A new consciousness of muscular
Frailty develops instantly and never
Completely resolves. Immobility
Is memorized like a prayer.

And one recovers, as in learning to love again
One almost inconceivably small step
At a time.

Jeremy Nobel, MD

The Almanac of Back Pain Treatments

Table of Contents

Author's Preface

"I know I have the body of a weak and feeble woman, but I have the heart and stomach of a king..." Queen Elizabeth I

When I began the search to find a cure for the debilitating back pain that was disrupting my life, I visited my family doctor, an orthopedic surgeon, a neurologist, a neurosurgeon, a rheumatologist, two osteopaths, an acupuncturist and two physical therapists. I tried a corset, acupuncture and the acupuncture diet, manipulation, various medications, bedrest, ultrasound, massage therapy, exercise programs, posture training, foot orthotics and positive thinking. I was advised to base my activity level on the pain and advised to ignore the pain. I was told that I should turn the pain over to God, that I should let myself get well and that my physical problem was a direct result of spiritual negativity. Friends insisted that osteopathy is the one answer, that acupuncture is the one answer and that chiropractic is the one answer. Diagnoses considered included muscle strain, degenerative disk disease, lupus (SLE), rheumatoid arthritis, somatic dysfunction, multiple sclerosis, prolapsed disks, piriformis syndrome and sacro-iliac joint dysfunction. My official diagnosis remains "low back pain".

One of the brightest days in the months of medical appointments and trial treatment was the day my family doctor, husband and I had a conference; we decided that the search for a diagnosis and cure had gone on long enough, that I have a disability which is probably permanent and that it was finally time to get on with my life. It was distressing to give up my career as a physical therapist, a vocation that had absorbed and defined me for years, but it was also an enormous relief to let go of the commitments I could no longer honor.

Chronic pain is with me daily, straining my physical and emotional resources. There is a struggle to maintain self-esteem, but also the emergence of new interests and new horizons. My back pain hasn't diminished in the years since its onset, but I consider myself to be a happy, productive person; it was impossible to be either when my only goal was to resume my former pain-free life. Now I can say "I'm fine!" and mean it.

While searching for answers to my own condition and in my professional research and experience, I have learned how controversial and complicated back pain is. My hope is that *The Almanac of Back Pain Treatments* can help those of you with acute, chronic or recurrent back pain find the ways to minimize your pain and proceed with your lives.

Introduction

"We are spending too much on treatments that are not proven and on diseases that aren't actually there." Charles Federspiel, PhD[6]

200 million of 250 million Americans will have back trouble before age 50;[1] in people younger than 45 it is the most frequent cause of disability. Back pain is the nation's most common musculoskeletal complaint, with 7 million disabled annually.[25] For 10 percent, or 20 million, the symptoms will become chronic. Back pain, the most expensive benign condition in America, costs up to $80 billion/year in lost wages and productivity,[2] plus many billions more in medical costs, disability claims, lawsuits and related expenses; no other affliction even comes close. Back problems are second only to upper respiratory infections for causing missed work and visits to the family doctor; they are responsible for the largest number of workers' compensation claims and up to 32 percent of disability payments.[25]

The phenomenal scope of this problem should mean that it is well understood. Unfortunately, the controversy surrounding the diagnosis and treatment of back pain proves otherwise. People with back pain frequently receive a variety of diagnoses, misdiagnoses or no diagnosis; finding the right treatment is often a matter of luck. Back pain may continue for months or years despite patients' best efforts and those of their heath care providers.

Diagnosis

"Early, accurate diagnosis is not absolutely essential." Mark Horwich, M.D.[16]
"The cause of chronic pain is a lack of diagnosis; truly effective, relieving treatment is unlikely without a diagnosis." William Wyatt, D.O. [34]

A patient who consults a GP, chiropractor, orthopedic surgeon, osteopath and alternative healer may get five different opinions as to the cause of his back pain. Each health practitioner seems to have a different explanation for a patient's symptoms. Many patients never receive a specific diagnosis and are classified as suffering from "low back syndrome".[31] The majority will never know the true underlying cause of their pain.[26] In fact, few back injuries can be traced to anatomical disorders and no medical test or examination technique can say what actually caused them.[22,30]

6

Although the principle obligation of a health care professional is to diagnose and treat pathology, there is often little to go on but the patient's report of pain. Health practitioners who treat back pain base treatment on their individualized views of what causes it and in which spinal structures the pain originates; the variation of opinions is staggering!

- *"Trauma is the most frequent cause of back pain, the main reason being that people are in poor physical condition."* [3]
- *"80 percent of back pain is caused by weak or tense muscles."* [33]
- *"50-70 percent of chronic symptoms are psychological in origin."* [5-A]
- *"The majority of lower-back pain actually originates in the sacral ligaments."* [8]
- *"An extremely high percentage of patients with pain have fascial problems."* [7]
- *"The majority of chronic disabling low back pain is from degenerative changes."* [17]
- *"Most neck, shoulder and back pain is due to Tension Myositis Syndrome."* [29]
- *"In 50 percent or more of back pain patients, the facet joint is the site of dysfunction."* [5-B]
- *"Chronic pain is caused by chronic guilt; back problems are due to a lack of feeling supported."* [15]
- *"Chronic sprain is probably the most common low back problem."* [21]
- *"Functional disorders of the musculoskeletal system called somatic dysfunctions are responsible for most (95 percent) back pain."* [4]
- *"90-95 percent of back pain is due to disks."* [5-C]
- *"Vertebral subluxations are found in every sick, malfunctioning body."* [20]
- *"Improper diet and lifestyle are the root of most of our medical problems."* [18]
- And from a British newspaper, *"There is a well-proven relationship between the number of cigarettes smoked and the likelihood the individual will have back problems."*

Obviously, the health care profession does not have a firm grasp on the condition which affects 80 percent of Americans. This is frightening for the person with back pain who wants to know immediately and with certainty

'What's wrong?' 'How serious is it?,' 'Will it get worse?,' and 'What do I do?' Most people assume that curative treatment can't begin until a health problem is accurately diagnosed. In the field of back pain, it is commonplace for treatment to be prescribed without a diagnosis or with a misdiagnosis.

Treatment

"Researchers say there's no clear-cut advantage of one kind of treatment over another." David Zinman [35]

"The vast majority of approaches to treating back pain patients have been found to be no better than no treatment at all." James McGavin, PT [24]

Given the lack of agreement concerning the diagnosis of back pain, it is not surprising that treatment for the condition is equally controversial. Treatment is often based on the philosophy and training of the practitioner rather than the patient's symptoms. Regardless of the treatment approach, 60-80 percent recover from an acute low back pain episode in three days to three weeks;[9] 90 percent recover within two months.[10] Most back aches get better despite treatment rather than because of it. When spontaneous recovery and medical intervention fail, back pain becomes chronic. Treatment continues, but it is often expensive, inappropriate and prescribed in response to the patient's pain level, not to address known pathology. The desperate wish for a quick fix also encourages non-conventional approaches which may be harmful. Many patients shop around and try, in the words of one neurosurgeon, "injections, stimulators, mechanical devices, and Rolfing, none of which can possibly have any curative effect."[14]

Another factor in treatment is the placebo effect; this is higher with back pain than with other kinds of pain. It is not unusual for 30 percent of people with back trouble to feel better after receiving therapy which has no possible pain relieving properties.[10,33] One explanation is that the body releases endorphins, (its own pain-killers), when people believe they are getting pain reducing treatment. Key factors are the patient's confidence in the healer and the healer's faith in the therapy. Unfortunately, the placebo effect is rarely long-lasting.

What with spontaneous recovery, the placebo effect and the changeable nature of pain, the claims made concerning the success of various treatments cannot be taken at face value. Although an army of "experts" claims to have found the answer for "most" back pain patients, this field has a dismal percentage of cure. If the following statements were all true, one would be at a loss to understand why so many Americans still suffer from recurrent or chronic back pain.

- *"I haven't seen any techniques that are so effective in reducing pain and restoring function as myofascial release."* [7]
- *"Mobilization and manipulation studies claim an 80 percent success rate."* [11]
- *"80 percent of low back pain patients get immediate relief with epidural blocks."* [32]
- *"In one study, the McKenzie approach revealed that 97 percent of patients improved over one week of treatment."* [24]
- *"With Meridian Therapy 40 percent were still free of complaints after one year and 30 percent were better."* [12]
- *"With microcurrent therapy, 95 percent of patients got pain relief and 82 percent were pain free within 10 treatments."* [27]
- *"90 percent of patients diagnosed with sacroiliac joint dysfunction without secondary factors obtained significant relief with manipulation."* [24]
- *"Radiofrequency facet denervation is more than 70 percent effective."* [28]
- *"95 percent were better or cured with manipulation under anesthesia preceded by a full eclectic regimen."* [19]
- *"In the YMCA's exercise program, 80 percent improve and 31 percent have pain completely eliminated."* [33]
- *"70-80 percent of those carefully screened for radicular symptoms benefit from surgery."* [9]

Although every technique helps some people with back pain, nothing works for everyone. Practitioners who diagnose the same problem and prescribe the same treatment regime for every patient don't help the majority of their patients. The onus is often on the patient to believe in a treatment in order for it to work, implying that those without optimistic attitudes will undermine the healer's efforts. However, it is unfair to expect people searching for relief to get their hopes up again and again. Practitioners of a specific philosophy shouldn't demand total commitment from a patient, but rather an open mind. The test of a treatment's success is what works in the long run.

Given the difficulty of receiving a firm diagnosis and the controversy surrounding the treatment of back pain, patients may despair of ever being pain-free. Fortunately, the people whose back pain signals a potentially serious disease have a good chance of being accurately diagnosed and effectively treated. The other 85-90 percent[6,13] are usually diagnosed with "low back syndrome" or with one of the conditions which falls into this category. These syndromes can be extraordinarily painful and limiting, but are not life-threatening. To provide the best chance for permanent pain relief and to avoid having the condition become chronic, it is crucial for patients to be evaluated by a professional who can relate specific symptoms to specific syndromes and then apply the appropriate therapy. Even if the primary pathology cannot be identified, treatment of symptoms can provide short-term relief. The response to symptomatic treatment may then further pinpoint the structures involved. The long-term goal is for function to improve and pain to decrease even if the specific origin of the problem is unknown.

The Almanac of Back Pain Treatments attempts to sort through the confusion of advice and promises, terminology and treatments that surround this subject. It explains the rationale behind the various therapies, giving individuals with back pain the knowledge that will let them make appropriate choices when looking for help. What works to the patient's advantage is to be as informed as possible about backs and what can happen to them. PART 1 looks at the normal and dysfunctional back and at the training and philosophy of health professionals. PARTS 2 and 3 provide an in depth examination of the traditional and alternative treatments for back pain, respectively. The final chapter, "Author's Recommendations," offers suggestions appropriate for everyone with back pain.

Using *The Almanac of Back Pain Treatments*

1) The information presented is based on the writings and research of practitioners in the field of back pain. Given the considerable controversy in this area, an attempt has been made to discuss opposing theories objectively and fairly.

2) In keeping with the attempt to present information objectively, the book is written in the third person. The exception is in sections which offer specific recommendations to "you", the person with back pain.

3) Certain sections in the book provide in depth or technical information on specific topics. These are boxed so that readers not interested in such detail can easily continue with the basic text.

4) For those unfamiliar with anatomical terms, the first chapter, "The Normal Back/The Painful Back", explains the normal anatomy and movement of the spine and the medical problems which can affect it. A complete glossary is included in Appendix A.

5) At the end of every chapter is a summary or overview of the information in that chapter, titled "Key Points".

6) Footnotes throughout the text refer to the numbered resources listed alphabetically at the end of each chapter. A complete bibliography is included in Appendix B.

7) People with acute back pain are "patients" during the diagnostic process and while receiving professional treatment. When a person's pain becomes chronic, the "patient" designation is no longer appropriate. In this book, people are referred to as "patients" only in the context of diagnosis and treatment.

8) *The Almanac of Back Pain Treatments* is written for the person with back pain, but is also appropriate for the health practitioner who treats back pain patients. Chapter 18 contains "Recommendations for Health Professionals."

Disclaimer

The purpose of *The Almanac of Back Pain Treatments* is to provide information regarding back pain and its treatment options. It should be used as a general guide and readers should tailor all information to their individual circumstances. **This book is in no way meant to take the place of an individualized evaluation and treatment plan from a qualified health professional.**

The author and Biddle Publishing Company have neither liability nor responsibility to any person with respect to any injury alleged to be caused directly or indirectly by the information contained in this book. If the reader does not wish to be bound by the above, the book may be returned to the publisher for a full refund.

Footnotes

1 Edward Abraham, *Freedom from Back Pain*
2 Henry Allen, "That Back's Gotta Come Out"

Introduction

PART 1 - STARTING THE SEARCH

Chapter 1 - The Normal Back/The Painful Back

Normal Anatomy of the Spine

"The thigh bone's connected to the hip bone, the hip bone's connected to the back bone, the back bone's connected to the neck bone, now hear the word of the Lord!" Source Unknown

"The back" functions as a single unit, but it is a complex structure composed of bones, joints, disks, muscles, ligaments, a spinal cord, nerve roots and all their connective and surrounding tissues. The back is shaped and supported by individual bony segments, the **vertebrae**; together they make up the vertebral or **spinal column**. The spinal column has four built-in curves, two concavities ("lordoses") of the low back and neck, and two convexities ("kyphoses") of the upper back and sacrum. These allow energy-efficient postural balance and serve a shock-absorbing role for the body. The spinal column is divided into five sections; the seven **cervical**, twelve **thoracic** and five **lumbar vertebrae** are separate bones, while the five **sacral vertebrae** are fused into one bone, the **sacrum**. The **coccyx**, or tailbone, is also one fused entity. [See Figure 1-1]

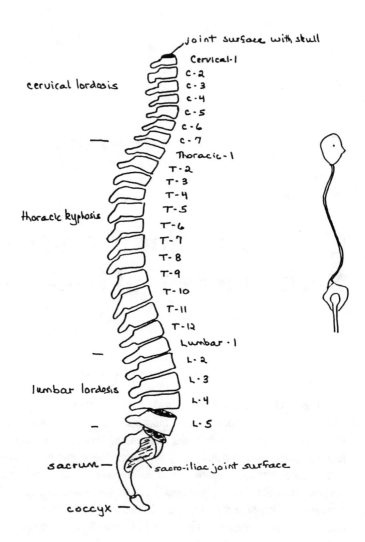

Figure 1-1. The spinal column, side view.

The spinal column is joined at the sacrum to the **pelvis**; this large bone is a ring composed of three sections (ilium, ischium and pubis). The sacro-iliac joints join the ilia of the pelvis to the sacrum; the pubic bones are connected anteriorly by strong fibrous tissue (the "pubic symphysis"). [See Figure 1-2]

Structures Joining Vertebra to Vertebra

(1) Intervertebral **disks** sit between the bodies of the vertebrae and provide cushioning and shock absorption; they have a tough fibrous outer ring (the "annulus fibrosis") and soft gelatin-like center (the "nucleus pulposis"). [See Figures 1-3 & 1-5]

(2) Each vertebra has seven bony projections or prominences – a spinous process posteriorly, two transverse processes laterally and four articular processes which extend up or down. [See Figures 1-4 & 1-5] **Facet joints** link the two superior articular processes of one vertebra to the two inferior articular processes of the vertebra above it. [See Figures 1-6 & 1-7] [See Box 1-1]

Facet Joints

Joints are interruptions in the skeleton where movement occurs; facet joints allow movement between the vertebrae. They are "synovial" type joints, as are most joints with detectable amounts of movement. Synovial joints are so-called because they are lined by a "synovial membrane" that produces fluid for lubrication and protection; a "joint capsule" surrounds and encloses the joint. Some synovial joints contain a "meniscus," a wedge-shaped crescent of solid tissue; one side of the meniscus attaches to the capsule and the free edge extends into the joint. [See Figure 1-8 C]

Box 1-1

---

(3) Structural reinforcement is provided by **ligaments**, tough and inelastic bands of tissue. The anterior and posterior "longitudinal ligaments" travel the length of the spine between vertebral bodies; with the shorter transverse ligaments, they tie adjacent vertebrae together. [See Figure 1-7]

(4) The primary function of **muscles** is not structural support or joining of bone to bone. Unlike ligaments, muscle tissue is elastic and, when stimulated by a nerve, contracts to pull two bony surfaces together. Muscles

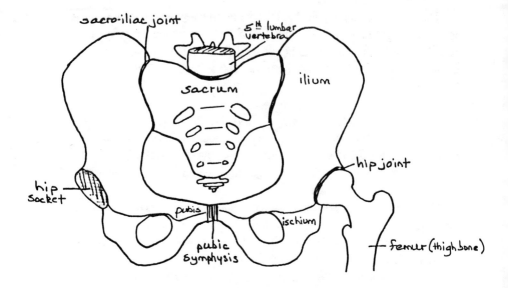

Figure 1-2. The pelvis and sacrum, front view.

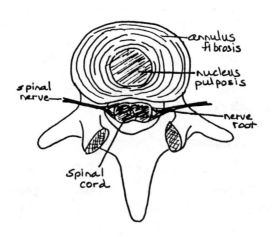

Figure 1-3. Vertebra with disk, spinal cord and nerve roots, top view.

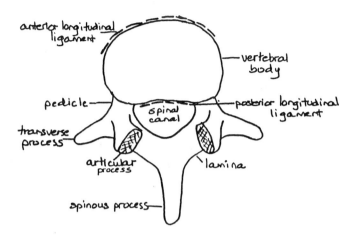

Figure 1-4. Vertebra with longitudinal ligaments, top view.

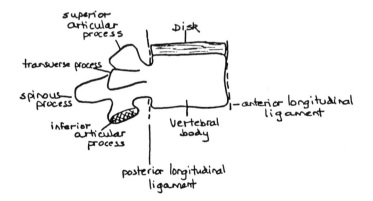

Figure 1-5. Vertebra with disk and longitudinal ligaments, side view.

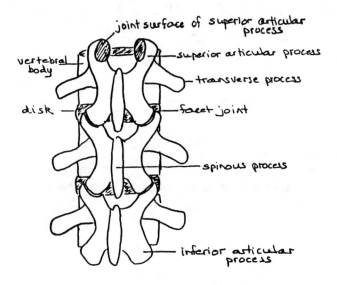

Figure 1-6. Section of the spinal column showing three vertebrae, back view.

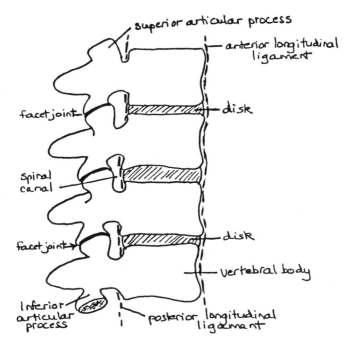

superior articular process

anterior longitudinal ligament

facet joint

disk

spinal canal

facet joint

disk

vertebral body

Inferior articular process

posterior longitudinal ligament

Figure 1-7. Section of the spinal column showing four vertebrae with disks and longitudinal ligaments, side view.

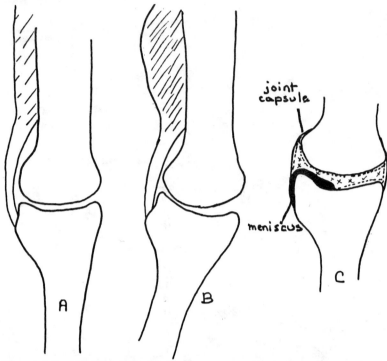

Figure 1-8. (A) Joint in extension with flexor muscle relaxed, side view. (B) Contraction and shortening of flexor muscle to move the joint into flexion. (C) Close-up side view of synovial joint with meniscus; dotted line represents synovial membrane and "x's" represent synovial fluid within the joint space.

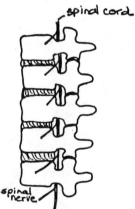

Figure 1-9. Section of the spinal column showing five vertebrae with disks, spinal cord and spinal nerves, side view.

provide strength for movement and postural holding. Some end in tendons, fibrous cords which attach muscle to bone. [See Figure 1-8 A & B]

(5) **Fascia** is connective tissue; it surrounds, permeates and joins all the structures and organs of the body. The brain and spinal cord are also covered by three fascia-type membranes, called "meninges." A liquid produced by the brain, "cerebrospinal fluid", fills the space between the two inner meninges to protect the brain and spinal cord.

Normal Movement of the Spine

"What a piece of work is man! . . . in form and moving how express and admirable!"
Shakespeare, *Hamlet*, Act 2, Scene 2

A passage called the **spinal canal** runs through the spinal column; within this spinal canal the **spinal cord** is located. The spinal cord consists of bundles of nerves which exit in pairs at each vertebra, carrying messages between the brain and body. [See Figures 1-3 & 1-9]

Sensation (including pain) travels from all parts of the body to the brain with information about the physical world. Specialized sensory nerves carry information about sight, taste, smell and sound. Nerve endings in the soft tissues of the body (the muscles, ligaments, and joint capsules) send the brain information about posture and movement. Feedback from these soft tissues plays a large role in both reflex and voluntary movement. These complex nervous system connections determine the response of the body's musculature to any stimulus, such as a shift in gravity, the decision to move or an injury.

Movement impulses travel in the opposite direction of sensation. Commands initiated in the brain travel down the spinal cord, out the nerve roots and along a nerve to the muscles, causing movement. When stimulated by a nerve impulse, muscles shorten and cause movement at joints by pulling two bony surfaces together. [See Figure 1-8 A & B] "Reflexes" are movements that happen so quickly they initially bypass the brain; a sensation travels inward only as far as the spinal cord, then immediately back to a muscle. For example, when someone touches a hot stove, her hand is jerked away before her brain can register pain.

Normal movement is limited by the shape, depth, type, and angle of joints, their ligamentous and muscular support and the presence of surrounding structures; due to all these factors different joints of the spine have different ranges of motion. The muscles that cross the small joints of the spine can cause movement in three planes.

- flexion/extension (bending and straightening)
- lateral flexion (bending away from the body's midline)
- rotation (twisting)

These facet joint movements are under voluntary control. Another kind of movement is called "joint play"; this refers to the small involuntary movements that occur within a joint in response to outside forces.

Normal Pain

"Pain is perception. Therefore all pain is in the brain." American Osteopathic Association[1]

Acute pain is a normal, protective response to alert the body to possible tissue damage. It is an unpleasant sensation, from discomfort to agony, caused by the stimulation of specialized nerve endings. Pain is primarily associated with physical injury, but since pain is a perception it may not be proportional or even directly related to an injury. The experience of hurting is a composite of physical, intellectual, emotional, motivational and situational reactions; factors other than tissue damage may directly affect the severity, tolerance and persistence of symptoms. In addition, pain does not necessarily correspond to the damaged area; it may move or change, and may or may not follow expected patterns of radiation. These are among the many reasons that pain may not be an accurate measure of the location and severity of an injury. They all need to be taken into consideration in the diagnosis and treatment of back pain.

Pain: An Unreliable Indicator of Pathology

1) Pain is highly subjective and influenced by emotional, intellectual and situational factors. A child may perceive the pain of a skinned knee differently in the presence of friends than in the company of his doting grandparents.

2) Accuracy of pain localization depends on nearness of the injury to the body surface. The pain from a rapped shin bone is well defined compared to the diffuse ache of an intestinal upset.

3) Pain perception does not necessarily correspond to the site of stimulation; pain can be referred to other structures. During a heart attack, severe pain may be felt down the left arm.

4) Different structures have different sensitivities to pain. [See Box 1-2]

Pain Sensitivity in Spinal Tissues

Some spinal structures are essentially without pain receptors or insensitive to pain; these include intervertebral disks, cartilage, vertebral bodies (unless invaded by cancer) and nerve roots. Pain responsive tissue (in the approximate order of sensitivity) includes the periosteum (outer covering of bone), joint capsules, synovial lining, ligaments (excepting the ligamentum flavum), subchondral bone (bone which lies beneath cartilage), tendons, nerves and nerve sheaths, fascia (connective tissue), cortical bone (bone which composes the outer layer of the shaft) and muscles.

In back dysfunction, the structures that usually give rise to pain are the anterior and posterior longitudinal ligaments, the outer covering of the nerve roots (the dura), the spinal muscles, the fascia of the muscles, the facet joints and the sacro-iliac joints.

Box 1-2

---

5) Severe pain in one structure can block pain from another structure. When someone stubs a toe, the pain from a headache is temporarily forgotten.

6) Pain is blocked by sensory stimulation. When an individual bangs her head, her tendency is to rub it. [See Box 1-3]

Gate Control Theory

Pain travels in small nerve fibers; it is usually blocked at the spinal cord by a steady volume of large fiber (sensory) impulses. When a strong enough painful stimulus occurs, the message of pain from the small pain fibers blocks the large fiber transmission to reach the brain and consciousness. Pain which would normally reach someone's awareness can in turn be blocked by increased levels of sensory stimulation. This view of pain perception is called gate control theory. It is discussed in Chapter 15 under "Acupuncture."

Box 1-3

---

7) Pain can radiate, following nerve, muscle or embryological patterns of distribution.[4] "Sciatica" is felt as pain down the back of the leg, but it usually indicates a problem in the lumbo-sacral spine.

8) Painful structures can increase pain perception or can block pain in other structures from the same embryological segment. [See Box 1-4]

Embryological Pain Patterns

Pain patterns associated with deep injury may be related to the embryological development of the musculoskeletal system. When one structure is injured, other structures which originated in the fetus from the same mass of tissue are affected. The results may include an embryological pattern of increased muscle tone, hyperactive reflexes and increased skin sensitivity.[4]

Box 1-4

---

9) Pain perception can depend on the temporal or spatial summation of stimuli. An individual can comfortably perform many repetitions of a specific exercise and then suddenly feel pain the next time the motion is repeated.

10) Pain is inconsistent and may change in location and severity. The ache of an arthritic hip may wax and wane throughout the day for no apparent reason.

11) Pain is strongly influenced by the "placebo effect," the relief of symptoms caused only by the belief that one is receiving a pain-relieving treatment. The placebo effect may work through the production of "endorphins," or natural pain killers. [See Box 1-5]

Endorphins

Endorphins are opiate-like derivatives produced by the brain which have a pain-killing effect on the body. The following are thought to stimulate the body to secrete endorphins. . .

- tissue damage
- laughter
- exercise
- manual therapy
- the placebo effect

Box 1-5

---

12) Pain can persist after the organic cause has been treated and thought to be corrected. A whiplash injury may result in chronic pain despite the fact that no evidence of tissue damage remains.

Spinal Dysfunction

"What we take for a cure is often just a momentary rally or a new form of the disease."
Duc Francois LaRochefoucauld

Back pain is a symptom present in a wide variety of health problems. Before assuming that a patient is one of the estimated 85-90 percent who falls into the "low back syndrome" category,[1,2] a physician may need to consider and rule out any number of conditions or diseases. These can be differentiated from the low back syndromes, because most can eventually be diagnosed through radiographic, laboratory or other tests. Examples are bone tumors, rheumatoid arthritis and spinal tuberculosis.

When the diagnosable diseases have been ruled out, some patients are left without a firm diagnosis; others are diagnosed with a syndrome involving pathology of one of the following spinal structures:

1) Intervertebral Disks - Commonly called slipped disks, this condition results when the inner part of the disk pushes through the outer fibers. If this causes a bulging, it is called a **prolapsed disk**; if a fragment pushes all the way through, it is a **ruptured disk**. Ruptured disks may or may not cause nerve root compression. [See Figure 1-10]

2) Facet Joints - The moveable joints linking the vertebrae are the facets.

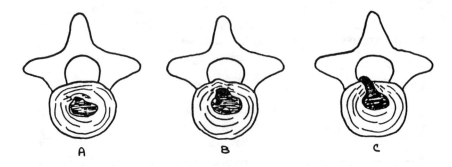

Figure 1-10. Increasingly severe levels of disk dysfunction, top view. (A) Tearing of inner annular fibers. (B) Tearing of inner and outer annular fibers with bulging of annulus into spinal canal. (C) Rupture of annular fibers with extrusion of nuclear material into the spinal canal.

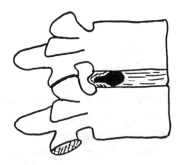

Section of vertebral column showing two vertebrae with a prolapsed disk bulging into the spinal canal and compressing the posterior longitudinal ligament, side view.

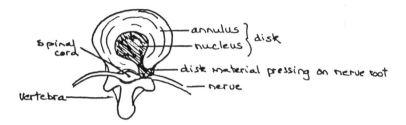

Vertebra, top view, with a ruptured disk compressing a nerve root.

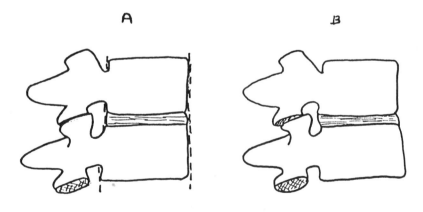

Figure 1-11. (A) Section of the spinal column showing two vertebrae, side view. (B) Subluxation of the facet joint causing narrowing of the spinal canal, with possible pinching of the soft tissues of the joint or entrapment of a spinal nerve against the vertebral body or disk.

A   B

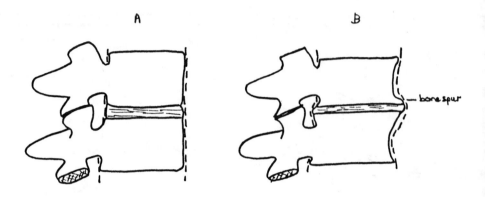

Figure 1-12. (A) Section of the spinal column showing two vertebrae, side view. (B) Spondylosis of spinal column (flattened and misshapen vertebral bodies, flattened disks, worn down and jammed fact joints, narrowed spinal canal, stretched ligaments and development of bone spurs).

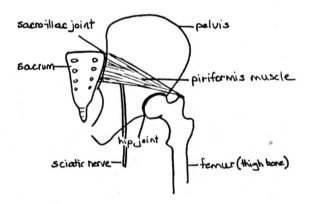

Figure 1-13. Pelvis, sacrum and thigh bone, back view, with piriformis muscle and sciatic nerve.

They are subject to a variety of **facet joint dysfunction** such as sprain, inflammation, arthritis and instability. One of these joints may also become displaced and jammed; when this happens the soft tissues of the joint can be pinched. This is called acute locked back syndrome. [See Figure 1-11]

3) Soft Tissue - The non-structural parts of the spine include muscles, tendons, ligaments and fascia. Injuries to muscles or ligaments are called **strains** and **sprains**, respectively. When a muscle stays tightened to protect itself or other structures, it is in **spasm**. The role of fascia, or connective tissue, as a primary site of back pain is gaining popularity, but is still controversial.

4) The Whole Spine - Degenerative disk disease, arthritis and degenerative disease of the spine are all terms used to describe the changes of aging; these affect vertebrae, disks, facet joints and soft tissues. The combination of these degenerative changes is called **spondylosis**. [See Figure 1-12]

5) Sacro-iliac Joints - The SI joint has limited movement, but it can become wedged and irritated, especially if it is excessively mobile to begin with. This syndrome is called **sacro-iliac joint dysfunction.**

6) Piriformis Muscle - This condition also involves soft tissue, but is localized to a specific muscle. If the piriformis muscle goes into spasm, it can compress the sciatic nerve, causing both localized and referred pain. This describes the **piriformis syndrome.** [See Figure 1-13]

There are many who think years of poor posture has the most dramatic impact on causing any of the six syndromes and is the chief culprit in most low back and neck problems. Poor posture is known to predispose disks, muscles and SI joints to injury and to speed the degenerative process of the spine.

The many structures of the spine are interrelated and injury to one can initiate pain and dysfunction in the others. Experts on back pain disagree widely on which is usually the site of the primary pathology. With six specific syndromes to choose from, one would expect that identifying the problem would be routine. Many factors complicate the issue. [See Box 1-2] Due to individual differences and the interrelatedness of spinal structures, pinpointing the site of primary pathology may be impossible. However, specific symptoms are usually associated with specific spinal structures; for many patients careful evaluation can lead to a definitive diagnosis. The more accurate the understanding of the symptoms, the easier it is to select the appropriate treatment approach. With or without a clear diagnosis, the doctor and patient must eventually decide on a plan to relieve and manage the patient's back pain.

---

1) Different distinct syndromes can yield the same symptoms.
2) Syndromes producing characteristic symptoms may occasionally present in an atypical way.
3) When facet joints are involved, the disk is affected and vice versa.
4) Muscle spasm may accompany spinal pain no matter what the cause.
5) Degenerative changes on x-rays may be unrelated to pain.
6) Radiating pain does not necessarily imply nerve root compression.
7) Pathology in one structure can cause mechanical problems in any weight-bearing joint.
8) Piriformis muscle spasm can cause sacro-iliac strain and vice versa.
9) Irritated tissue in a sclerotome (deep tissues innervated by the same spinal nerve) can cause irritation in all tissues of that sclerotome.
10) Sclerotomes and dermatomes (skin area innervated by the same spinal nerve) do not correspond exactly.

Box 1-2

Key Points - The Normal Back

The back is a complex unit made up of vertebrae, disks, facet joints, sacro-iliac joints, ligaments, muscles and connective tissue. Each structure assists in one or both of the dual functions of the spine – stability and movement. Back pain can be the result of dysfunction in any one of these structures; diagnosis and treatment requires an understanding of their normal functions and interrelationships.

Pain is a normal protection mechanism of the body which signals potential tissue damage. However, pain is not a reliable guide to the location or extent of an injury. Identification of the primary site of pain can be difficult, even impossible. Every evaluation and treatment of patients with back pain must be individualized.

Footnotes

1 American Osteopathic Association, informational literature
2 *The Back Letter*, Vol. 4, No. 3
3 Richard DonTigny, "Function and Pathomechanics of the Sacroiliac Joint"
4 Stanley Paris, *The Spine*

Chapter 2 - The Doctors

Medical Doctors

"It is not the business of the doctor to say that we must go to a watering place; it is his affair to say that certain results to health will follow if we do go to a watering place." Gilbert Keith Chesterton

MDs are required to complete four years of undergraduate education, four years of medical school, one year of internship, state licensure and continuing education credits - just to practice as GPs (General Practitioners). Most then add a two to seven-year residency and take national boards to become specialists. MDs have the whole of modern technology and science available to them for diagnosis and treatment; standard Western medicine is usually considered the only realistic option for preserving the lives of patients with certain diseases or injuries.[13]

A patient's family doctor, (usually a Family Practice or Internal Medicine specialist), may refer the patient to another physician with in depth training in a specific area. There are a variety of specialists who may be involved in the care of back pain patients.

Specializing Physicians

Neurosurgeons - referral for patients with clear signs of nerve or nerve root compression

Neurologists - referral with the presence of neurologic signs and symptoms other than those indicative of nerve root compression

Physiatrists (doctors of physical medicine) - referral for those with back pain related to non-surgical orthopedic or movement dysfunction

Rheumatologists - referral with signs of systemic rheumatoid disease or arthritis

Orthopedic surgeons - referral when x-rays show gross structural abnormalities or traumatic injury

Psychiatrists - referral when pain reports seem grossly exaggerated or abnormal, coping skills are inadequate or emotional factors are interfering with diagnosis and treatment

When radiographic and blood test studies are negative and there are no clear signs that make referral to a specialist appropriate, the patient probably falls into the "low back syndrome" category. This vague diagnosis is a frustration for both patient and doctor. In this case, the role of the primary care physician is to present the therapeutic options available and recommend a course of action, which the patient is free to accept or reject. As time passes, a review of the situation can lead to alternative recommendations. Doctor and patient work best as a team in the management of the patient's overall health needs.

Criticism of MDs

Physicians are often criticized for providing little help to patients with back pain. Complaints include the following:
- the expense and brevity of an office visit
- a diagnosis based only on x-rays
- a condescending attitude
- an approach that treats only the spine, ignoring the whole person
- an approach that treats only through the suppression of symptoms, ignoring the spiritual/emotional bases of pain

Illness does not merely affect the body; a person is influenced by culture, society, relationships, the perceived future, the roles one functions in, spiritual beliefs, intelligence and emotional makeup.[4] As Dr. Eric Cassel writes in the *The New England Journal of Medicine*,

"It is not possible to treat sickness as something that happens solely to the body without thereby risking damage to the person. An anachronistic division of the human condition into what is medical (having to do with the body) and what is nonmedical (the remainder) has given medicine too narrow a notion of its calling. Because of this division, physicians may, in concentrating on the cure of bodily disease, do things that cause the patient as a person to suffer." [4]

In the treatment of back pain, the family physician often lacks experience in approaches beyond conservative, symptomatic measures, (rest, heat, medications, etc.). What the family physician can do, however, is look for the diagnosable diseases that affect about 10-15 percent of back pain patients.[2,8] Practitioners who offer alternatives to standard Western medicine can miss the signs and symptoms that make referral to the appropriate medical consultant crucial. A physician is the best professional to find or rule out serious illness. A medical doctor can also offer the back pain patient an appropriate referral to a practitioner with the ability to provide individualized evaluation and treatment.

Therapies Through Physician Referral

"paindemons / skewer me / to the floor again / a quivering heap / lying in a quagmire / of tears and tangled hair; / face grotesque / with grimaces; / lips blue / around gritting teeth; / cursing, / fighting back, / doing the damned / exercises- / i want my arm back!" Ardeana Hamlin, "Physical Therapy - First Sessions"

Physical Therapy

Physicians often refer back pain patients to Physical Therapy. PTs have a four-year Bachelor of Science or a graduate degree in Physical Therapy and take a state registry exam to become licensed. In some states PTs are now able to practice through direct access, without physician referral. Goals of PT are to. . .

- identify dysfunction (increased, decreased or abnormal movement)
- pinpoint affected structures
- relieve pain
- restore function, and
- prevent recurrence.

Although physical therapy is often equated with hot packs and whirlpools, these modalities are primarily used to prepare a patient for the more essential programs aimed at the restoration of normal movement.

PTs often specialize in the treatment of specific disabilities, but they are not certified as specialists. This means that a doctor's prescription is good for any registered therapist, but that therapists are not proficient in every therapeutic technique. The most effective PTs are those who have a well-rounded view of back pain and who don't become over committed to one philosophy.[16] In addition to treating the specific dysfunction, PTs also need to look at the overall status of the patient and address posture, body mechanics, physical conditioning, etc.

Patients with back pain all used to be treated with the same regime, ("Williams flexion exercises"), but it is now widely recognized that each program needs to be individualized. Although PTs do not diagnose disease, they should be proficient at diagnosing dysfunction. A physical therapist who is familiar with the range of approaches for "low back syndrome", (Williams versus McKenzie exercise programs, mobilization techniques, identification of Sacro-iliac Joint Dysfunction, etc.), has the best chance of localizing a patient's problem and providing successful treatment.

Occupational Therapy

The educational requirements for occupational therapists are similar to those of PTs – a four year B.S. or graduate degree with state registration and continuing education credits. Occupational therapy has traditionally not played as large a role as physical therapy in the treatment of back pain, but this is changing. OTs have expertise in a large variety of developmental and rehabilitative services; they are part of the team at pain clinics and involved in the return to work of patients injured on the job. OTs may provide therapy for pain coping, pain management, the psychological complications of pain, work hardening, evaluation of functional capacity and adaptation of the home or work environment.

Kinesiotherapy

Kinesiotherapists work under the auspices of a physiatrist, (a doctor of physical and rehabilitative medicine). They are commonly employed in the Veteran's Administration system, but also work in the private sector. KTs have a bachelor's degree and 1,000 hours of clinical training; they take a national certification exam and participate in continuing education. Areas of expertise include physical fitness training, exercise, disabled driver training and acute and chronic patient care.[7] In VA hospitals where there is a shortage of physical therapists, KTs have been accused of performing treatments beyond the scope of their training. Gait training, therapeutic exercise and evaluation of strength and range of motion are treatments more appropriately carried out by a PT.[17]

Osteopathic Doctors

"The DO has an advantage over the MD in that the DO is trained in manipulative therapy." Bob Jones[9]

"During the last decade, osteopathic schools have deemphasized manipulation." Randolph Kessler, PT & Darlene Hertling, PT[10]

Osteopathy differs from general medicine in its emphasis on the role of the musculoskeletal system in health and disease and in its use of spinal manipulation. Osteopaths also take a holistic approach to medicine, focusing on the patient as a whole, versus a specific illness. Educational requirements include three years at the college level, a four-year degree program, one year of internship, state licensure and continuing education; 45 percent of osteopaths go on for specialization.[1] DOs can now prescribe drugs, do surgery and provide a whole range of medical services. In fact, DOs and MDs have come to work more and more closely together; many osteopaths practice medicine in almost identical fashion to MDs and refer patients to specializing physicians and therapists. Manipulation, the distinctive feature and the original basis of the profession, is currently being deemphasized in osteopathic schools. [See Box 2-1]

The Basis of Osteopathy

In 1874 Andrew Still founded Osteopathy, a medical approach based on the premise that "body structure governs function and disturbances of structure lead to disturbances of function."[15] The musculoskeletal system, in addition to providing framework and support, has a major influence on the body's ability to maintain wellness. When this structure is healthy, the circulatory and nervous systems carry maintenance and repair capabilities to the rest of the body; the body is then able to be self-regulating and self-healing in the face of disease. Improper muscle functioning can impede blood and nerve supply, causing illness in other parts of the body. Manipulation of the musculoskeletal components can return the whole body to health through its effects on the circulatory and nervous systems. Some osteopaths recommend regular manipulation as a preventative measure for greater well-being and lowered susceptibility to illness in general.[9]

Box 2-1

Osteopathic Diagnosis: Somatic Dysfunction

While more and more DOs now work as specialists in a hospital setting, there are still many osteopaths whose practice consists primarily of treatment through manipulation. They believe that close to 95 percent of back pain is caused by what they call "somatic dysfunctions".[18] These are functional, or nonstructural, disorders of the musculoskeletal system; they are associated with pain, muscle spasm, structural malalignment and impaired mobility. Because unwellness is reflected throughout the body, illness or injury of any structure or system can cause somatic dysfunction. Once present, somatic dysfunctions deplete energy, lower resistance and can produce problems in the internal organs. In other words, a somatic dysfunction may . . .

(1) trigger disease in the rest of the body

(2) perpetuate disease by interfering with recovery

(3) indicate the presence of internal disease, or

(4) once initiated, can itself become a secondary disease, remaining even after the precipitating factor is gone.

Somatic dysfunction can only be diagnosed through palpation (hand-on examination) of musculoskeletal structures and the careful observation of movement. Although evaluation and manipulative treatment focus on the muscles, the final effects occur within the nervous system, affecting the whole body. Manipulation restores function through relaxation and lengthening of muscles; this then decreases the abnormal sensory input to the nervous system. The body is then able to regain a normal, balanced state so that unwell parts of the body can repair themselves. Chronic pain or illness results when somatic dysfunction is not properly diagnosed and treated.[18]

A recent study of patients receiving osteopathic manipulation produced the following results. The treatment significantly benefitted some patients whose pain had lasted 2-4 weeks, but did not benefit those with shorter or longer episodes of pain. In addition, after 4 weeks of treatment no advantage could be detected for those patients who had received osteopathic manipulation compared to patients who received no manipulation.[3] Manipulation as a treatment for back pain is controversial; its rationale, benefits and risks are discussed in Chapter 12, "Manual Therapy."

Chiropractors

"Vertebral subluxations [asymmetries] *are found in every sick, malfunctioning body."* John Langone[11]
"Asymmetry of the human body is not the exception, but the rule." James McGavin, PT[12]

Chiropractic and osteopathy are often confused; both emphasize the importance of the musculoskeletal system in overall health, both developed in the late 1800's, both have names that are not self-explanatory and both use manipulation to treat disease.[9] Chiropractors, however, are not licensed to provide a full range of medical services; they are limited to diagnosis and treatment of structural changes in the spinal column. The concern of the profession is the relationship between impaired movement of vertebrae and the nervous system, and its effect on health.[5] Chiropractic has both vehement advocates and critics; it is considered by medical and osteopathic physicians to fall considerably short of comprehensive medicine. Some consider this an asset and view chiropractic as a profession which offers patients safer or less toxic alternatives to prescription medications and surgery. [See Box 2-2]

The Basis of Chiropractic

Founded by Daniel Palmer in 1895, chiropractic is based on the "Law of the Nerve"; this states that the body has all the necessary components for health and that disease occurs when nerve impulses are reduced or changed. Misaligned spinal bones interfere with the normal pattern of nerve impulses, decreasing the body's efficiency and resistance to infection. Loss of alignment of the vertebral column can result from such factors as gravitational stress, strains, postural or movement asymmetry, developmental defects or nervous system irritations. Since spinal malalignments interfere with nerve and blood supply to the rest of the body, these off-centerings of the vertebrae can then cause disease. Once produced they become the focus of sustained pathology. For this reason, chiropractors treat all human ailments through manipulation of the spine.[13]

Box 2-2

Chiropractic Diagnosis: Vertebral Subluxation

A "subluxation" is the name for an off-centering or malalignment of one vertebra relative to other vertebrae. Subluxations are functional defects - they may not show on a standard x-ray but are apparent through movement limitations. Unlike osteopaths, chiropractors palpate for vertebral displacement rather than decreased mobility. To further pinpoint subluxations, chiropractors take full body x-rays in the positions in which the patient's pain is present; x-rays of the relaxed body in the lying down position are not useful because at rest the effects of muscle contraction and gravity are eliminated and subluxations are least in evidence. In addition to x-rays and palpation, chiropractors may use a "thermograph," a diagnostic technique which measures spinal heat. A subluxation interferes with blood supply, causing a drop in temperature; cold spots may also result from nerve compression, muscle spasm or areas of tenderness. Thermographs also identify hot spots resulting from inflamed nerves and muscles.

Variation Among Chiropractors

All chiropractors agree that subluxation plays a role in disease, but there are two schools of chiropractic thought. "Straights" stick to the "Law of the

Nerve" and treat all disease with manipulation; assessment is based solely on subluxations so they see no need to diagnose disease.[5] "Mixers" tend to be more liberal, treating other joints, using other treatment forms and making more modest claims. Mixers are more apt to accept the limitations of manipulation and supplement it with a variety of modalities - heat, cold, water, electricity, vitamin therapy, mechanical devices, diet, exercise, massage, psychotherapy, acupuncture or any combination of these.

Today, the straight chiropractic faction is said by some to be hurting the profession; it is seen as irresponsible to claim to provide primary health care and yet see no need to diagnose. There are only two colleges of straight chiropractic in the U.S. and these are not recognized by the accrediting agency for chiropractic schools.[5] The chiropractic profession seems to be moving away from its original rigid philosophy. Many chiropractors no longer claim to treat all diseases through spinal adjustments. Subluxations are more broadly defined to be: neurological or circulatory involvement due to (1) structural displacement of vertebrae or (2) abnormal function (movement) in a spinal segment. The mechanisms involved are recognized to often go beyond a simple pinching of a nerve by a displaced vertebra.[5]

Opposition to Chiropractic
Much criticism is leveled at chiropractic, and it focuses on a variety of concerns.

1) **Education.** Past standards for education were dreadful - in 1942 one could still purchase a chiropractic degree through the mail. Admission requirements were low, teachers and science courses inferior, and a 1972 study concluded that "deficiencies were too pervasive to permit an adequate educational experience."[6] Chiropractic education has improved since then; requirements now call for two years of college and four years of professional school. Diagnosis is now in the curriculum, but without hospital training or residency, chiropractic students (and instructors) don't see the range of diseases that DOs and MDs do. This means that the ability to diagnose contraindications to treatment is still a weak area; "straights" don't diagnose at all.[5] There is also minimal training in pharmacology; this is relevant because many chiropractors prescribe vitamins and discourage the use of drug therapy.[6]

2) **Radiation.** 90 percent of chiropractic patients are x-rayed, (compared with 3 percent who see MDs).[6] Chiropractors are looking for structural

malalignment to treat. However, slight postural shifts in standing can cause asymmetry during filming, giving the appearance of a minor subluxation. In addition, asymmetry exists in normal, pain-free spines. Chiropractors often take x-rays in full side-bending; people normally don't function in this extreme range, so these x-rays don't represent the spine in its typical position.[14] Some feel the massive radiation used by chiropractors is unwarranted and is used primarily to impress patients.[6]

3) **Philosophy.** Using manipulation to treat all diseases through its effects on the nervous system is the original philosophy of chiropractic; such effects are inconsistent and inconclusive when subjected to clinical trials.[15] The only parts of the nervous system accessible to manipulation are the 26 pairs of spinal nerves. This leaves 12 pairs of cranial nerves, 5 pairs of sacral nerves, the spinal cord, brain and parasympathetic nervous system which cannot be affected by manipulative treatment. Furthermore there is no scientific evidence that minor subluxations impinge on spinal nerves. Even some advocates of chiropractic now state, *"No responsible chiropractor today claims to cure organic disease through adjustments of the spine."*[5]

4) **Risk.** Doctors should weigh risks against benefits before initiating treatments with possible side-effects. When chiropractors use manipulation as a universal therapy, this is not a consideration, and a patient may be harmed by inappropriate treatment. 4 percent of patients in one study suffered direct injuries from chiropractic, from increased pain to serious nerve damage.[6] There is even a slight risk of stroke associated with cervical adjustments.[5] Chiropractic is also blamed for keeping patients from appropriate, timely medical treatment in cases of serious illness.

There is no question that chiropractors help some back pain patients, but the reasons are highly controversial. Many people visit their chiropractors regularly, claiming significant relief from minor back pain and stiffness. Others go regularly for general health maintenance. One author states, *"Preventive treatment for children is important, and regular check-ups are recommended."*[13]

Consumer Reports, an organization whose purpose is impartial testing of products and services, has studied the chiropractic profession. Its editors have written that chiropractic is a significant hazard to many patients and recommends the following for those who pursue this approach:[6]

1) Limit it to appropriate muscular complaints.
2) Refuse x-rays and vitamin therapy.

3) By-pass chiropractic altogether for the treatment of children.

4) Avoid chiropractors who make claims about miraculous cures, who never make referrals to other health practitioners and who use scare tactics about what may happen if treatment is delayed.

Manipulation's rationales, benefits and risks are discussed in Chapter 12, "Manual Therapy".

Key Points - The Doctors

Back pain patients are often confused about which type of doctor to consult. Medical doctors, osteopaths and chiropractors all have advocates and critics. The education that MDs and DOs receive is now very similar and includes years of hospital training. MDs often refer patients to specializing physicians or to physical therapy for treatment. Chiropractic evaluation and treatment is limited to structural changes in the spinal column. Both chiropractors and osteopaths emphasize the role of the musculoskeletal system in health and disease, and both treat back pain with manipulation. Osteopaths manipulate to correct somatic dysfunctions and chiropractors to correct vertebral subluxations.

This chapter covers the educational backgrounds, philosophies, methods of treatment and criticisms of medical doctors, osteopaths and chiropractors. It is recommended that in order to rule out potentially serious conditions, patients consult physicians with access to the full range of diagnostic services.

Footnotes

1 American Osteopathic Association, informational literature
2 *The Back Letter*, Vol. 4, No. 3
3 *The Back Letter*, Vol. 4, No. 9
4 Eric Cassell, "The Nature of Suffering and the Goals of Medicine"
5 David Chapman-Smith, "Chiropractic - A Referenced Source of Modern Concepts, New Evidence"
6 Consumer Reports Books, *Health Quackery*
7 Terry Dimick, "Kinesiotherapist Responds"
8 Richard DonTigny, "Function and Pathomechanics of the Sacroiliac Joint"
9 Bob Jones, *The Difference a D.O. Makes*
10 Kessler & Hertling, *Management of Common Musculoskeletal Disorders*
11 John Langone, *Chiropractors: A Consumer's Guide*

Chapter 2

12 James McGavin, "The McKenzie Approach to Spinal Pain"
13 Mills & Finando, *Alternatives in Healing*
14 Stanley Paris, "Physical Signs of Instability"
15 Stanley Paris, *The Spine*
16 David Reese, "Keep PT the Art That It Is"
17 Ellen Strickland, "Trouble with KTs"
18 William Wyatt, DO, literature for patients

Chapter 3 - Comparing Health Care Providers

"Fashions in therapy may have some justifications; fashions in diagnosis have none."
Robert Herrick

Comparing the Doctors

"Illness is the most heeded of doctors: to goodness and wisdom we only make promises; pain we obey." Marcel Proust

Some medical doctors, osteopaths and chiropractors have a tendency to look down on the other two professions, each believing their own approach to be the most enlightened. Their relative successes in eliminating back pain, as rated by the Klein and Sobel survey of back pain patients, are equally unimpressive.[6]

percentage providing dramatic long-term help
- family doctors - 8 percent
- osteopaths   - 7 percent
- chiropractors (manipulation only) - 5 percent
                (total care) - 14 percent

percentage ineffective or making patient feel worse
- family doctors - 66 percent
- osteopaths   - 57 percent
- chiropractors (manipulation only) - 44 percent
                        (total care) - 44 percent

Physiatrists (MDs specializing in physical and rehabilitation medicine) have more success than any of these doctors, with 33 percent providing dramatic long-term relief and only 14 percent ineffective or making the patient feel worse. Physical therapists also score higher with ratings of 34 percent and 27 percent, respectively. Physiatrists treat patients with a broad range of back conditions. They use physical modalities and exercise in addressing movement problems and work closely with physical therapy. Unfortunately, physiatrists are few in number, practicing mostly in large cities.[6]

For patients with negative x-rays and blood tests, a common frustration with medical doctors is their unwillingness to provide a concrete diagnosis. Negative diagnostic tests may be interpreted as meaning that nothing serious is wrong. The patient may be asked about stress, causing him to fear that the doctor thinks the pain "is all in my head". Osteopaths and chiropractors, on the other hand, know exactly what's wrong, (somatic dysfunction and subluxation, respectively), and how to treat it, (manipulation). Finding a practitioner who can confidently pinpoint the problem comes as a great relief - unless the treatment is ineffective. Unfortunately, manipulation alone seldom provides long-term relief.[2,4,6]

It is important to remember that pain relief is only one goal when seeking medical help; diagnosis is the other. The people whose back pain indicates serious illness can eventually be firmly diagnosed through laboratory or radiographic tests and are likely to receive effective treatment for their conditions. Other back patients may not get pain relieving therapy from their physicians, but may receive significant help in other areas. Their physicians can rule out disease, make referrals for effective treatment, offer emotional support and assist in the development of a plan for pain management.

The common denominator for success among the three types of doctors seems to be the following:[6]

1) an ability and willingness to explore the situations that increase pain and relate symptoms to specific spinal structures

2) the application of appropriate, individualized treatment based on the

results of the evaluation

3) consideration of the patient's daily living habits and general health, with recommendations concerning posture, body mechanics, exercise, etc.

or

4) making a referral to a practitioner who has these skills.

Traditional Versus Alternative Medical Approaches

"Care more for the individual patient than for the special features of the disease." Sir William Osler

The treatments for back pain are many and their classification is not always clear. The approaches which are most commonly and traditionally used to treat people with back problems can very generally be said to target the back versus promoting overall health. These methods also tend to fall into the realm of standard Western medicine and to be administered by registered health professionals.

There is much talk about alternative ways to treat health problems; usually what is meant is alternatives to surgery and prescription medications. It is frequently stated that Western medicine treats only symptoms, ignoring their causes, or treats only diseases, ignoring the patient. Many alternative approaches are "holistic"; they emphasize that the physical, mental, emotional and spiritual sides of a person must all be addressed in treatment. Every person is considered to be an integral part of the creative force of nature and the universe; health involves an increasing awareness of that universal energy.[5]

"Everything is one; there are no accidents. Labelling anything as a chance happening resulting from either randomness, coincidence or luck merely exposes our ignorance of the interrelationships that brought it about."[3]

Holistic practitioners place great emphasis on removing the obstacles, (physical, psychological or spiritual), that prevent the body from healing itself. Patients are responsible for their own health and disease;[5] with the support and guidance of the health practitioner, they are helped to make the changes in their lives that will promote recovery. Other concepts common to many alternative and holistic approaches include the uninterrupted flow of energy through the body, balance among the various influences on the body, and the role of the body's connective tissue in dysfunction.

These less traditional treatments are becoming more popular; they are administered by a variety of practitioners, many who are licensed professionals and some who are self-proclaimed and unregulated. Alternative healers do help some back pain patients; the ones who best serve the whole person are able to accept the following concepts:

1) Standard Western medicine is not merely the pharmacological or surgical repression of symptoms.

2) Patients should not be led to expect miracles from alternative approaches, then held responsible if the treatment is unsuccessful.

3) Every patient and every health problem is different; a single treatment approach is unable to help every patient.

4) Every person has a right to his or her own spiritual philosophy; holistic professionals who provide physical treatment should beware of tying spiritual/world view counseling to clinical techniques.[1,5]

The medical profession is often unwilling to take alternative approaches seriously. On the other hand, many holistic practitioners condemn traditional medicine as uncaring, ineffective or harmful. A rigid or defensive attitude on the part of any health practitioner is unfortunate. It is in a patient's best interest to feel comfortable exploring a variety of approaches to determine which will be most effective. Some people will be helped by conventional approaches and some by alternatives, and probably many by a combination. Whatever treatment can relieve a patient's pain and dysfunction, be it visualization or back exercises, should be supported by the practitioner, be he Rolfer or neurologist.

Key Points - Comparing Health Care Providers

It is recommended that to rule out potentially serious conditions, patients with back pain consult physicians with access to the full range of diagnostic services. Survey results indicate that all three types of doctors are unsuccessful in providing long-term, dramatic help for most back pain patients. Success is highest for those professionals who can individualize diagnosis and treatment and address the patient's overall health needs.

Traditional and alternative approaches to the treatment of back pain are many and varied. Health care providers are often unwilling to objectively consider therapies outside their own area of expertise; many are defensive about perceived criticism and unable to admit their limitations. Individualization of diagnosis and treatment means that practitioners put the patient's welfare ahead of a rigid philosophy of health care.

Footnotes

1 Benanti & Ellis, "Holistic Medicine a 'Crisis' for PTs"
2 Rene Cailliet, *Low Back Pain Syndrome*
3 Annemarie Colbin, *Food and Healing*
4 Richard DiFabio, "Clinical Assessment of Manipulation and Mobilization of the Lumbar Spine"
5 Nina Kim, "Holistic Medicine Requires Different World View"
6 Klein & Sobel, *Backache Relief*

PART 2 - TRADITIONAL TREATMENTS FOR BACK PAIN

Chapter 4 - Conservative Treatment

"Get some books and go to bed and rest for anywhere from a few days to a few weeks." Ben Benjamin[3] / *"Bed rest must be complete, continuous, correct and sufficiently prolonged; bathroom privileges must be curtailed."* Rene Cailliet, MD 1962[4]
"When prolonged, bedrest may be the most significant iatrogenic* cause of disability in spinal patients." James McGavin, PT[11] / *"There is no indication for prolonged bedrest as being beneficial in treating the acute low back pain patient. The vague advice of a week to ten days bedrest has actually proven to be not only useless but detrimental."* Rene Cailliet, MD, 1988[5]
* iatrogenic - caused by medical treatment

Patients with back pain, whatever the diagnosis, are advised to try conservative treatment before invasive procedures are considered. Conservative treatment traditionally means bedrest, heat, massage, traction, medications and/or mechanical supports such as corsets or cervical collars. When pain permits, patients are then advised to start an exercise/posture/body mechanics program. The fundamentals of proper use of the back are taught in "back school," a class offered by many physical therapy departments. In the long run, patients are advised to make changes in life style, such as losing weight and either slowing down or increasing activity level. The research that supports these various approaches is unclear regarding importance and applicability to different kinds of back pain. In researching treatments for back pain patients, compliance is hard to measure, there are long-term drop-outs, diagnoses are ambiguous and the outcome used for measurement varies among studies.

Bedrest

For the first few days of an acute back pain episode, when virtually all motion is impossible, a patient should probably bow to the inevitable and lie down. One to two days in bed can decrease pain and inflammation and provide a psychological break - but the less time spent on bedrest the better. The vague advice of a week to 10 days of bedrest is still handed out for any back complaint despite the fact that it has been proven to be not only useless, but detrimental.[5] In addition to harmful systemic effects, inactivity causes a loss of calcium in the bones, delay of tissue healing and a 3 percent loss of muscle strength/day. Prolonged bedrest can also cause psychological depression and dependency and interfere with return to work; it may make a worker more injury prone due to his deconditioned status.[3]

The idea behind bedrest is to remove the effects of gravity, allowing the antigravity muscles to rest and recover. However, the effects of muscle spasm, (pain, decreased blood flow and the accumulation of toxins in the tissues), can actually be increased by immobility. Moreover, there is no evidence that activity during the acute phase of back pain increases tissue damage. Avoidance of excessive activity and exercise is advisable, but total bedrest is not essential even for disk protrusion; rest should be alternated with gentle activity. With a disk rupture, a maximum of a week of bedrest may be necessary.[7] [See Box 4-1]

Positioning for Bedrest

The "proper" position to assume in bed is the one which is most comfortable and permits rest.[5] Backlying with knees and hips flexed is the traditionally recommended position; lying flat on back or stomach is thought to contribute to excessive lordosis. However, maintaining or even exaggerating a lordosis is beneficial for the patient with disk problems. In addition to backlying on a firm mattress with a cushion under the knees, a position which puts minimum pressure on the spine is sidelying with a pillow between the knees; the pillow keeps the spine from twisting, the top flexed leg from slipping forward, and the lower leg relatively extended. Positions which maintain a lumbar lordosis include stomachlying with a firm mattress, backlying with a lumbar roll or sidelying as described. Patients on "total" bedrest are supposed to eliminate or minimize all weight-bearing, but usually bedrest should be interspersed with short periods of walking about.

Box 4-1

In summation, there is no indication for prolonged or total bedrest in treating back pain. Early activity must be ensured; recommendations for total rest and avoidance of activity should not be prescribed.[5] Bedrest lacks scientific justification and its well-known detrimental effects when prolonged may be a significant contributor to chronic disability in back patients.[11]

Physical Agents

Physical modalities alone, (heat, ice, ultrasound, electricity), cannot cure low back problems; however, they may be effective in controlling pain so that treatment of the dysfunction can begin. They should be considered as a means of assisting active movement.[7] Benefits of heat, (hot packs, heat lamps, ultrasound, diathermy, etc.), are thought to be increased circulation and relaxation of muscle spasm to promote healing. However, unless muscle spasm is the primary cause of pain, treatment with heat and ultrasound is not useful and may increase inflammation. Soothing as it is, it may even reinforce psychological dependence.[12] Icing versus heat is now recognized as the treatment of choice in the acute stages of an injury to reduce inflammation; two to three minute ice massages may be more effective than an ice pack.[1]

A common technique used by professionals for pain inhibition is "Transcutaneous Electrical Nerve Stimulation," or TENS. A patient using a TENS unit glues or sticks electrodes on certain skin sites; a mild electrical current, either steady or pulsed, stimulates the skin in order to inhibit pain in the back. The electrical stimulation blocks the transmission of pain impulses; (the mechanism involved is described in Chapter 15 under "Acupuncture"). The maximum current which is not unpleasant should be used. TENS units are given to patients to use on their own.

Some patients using TENS report needing shorter periods of stimulation and getting longer periods of relief; this suggests that pain inhibition may have increasingly long-lasting effects.[16] However, TENS is not always successful. A study reported in *The New England Journal of Medicine* states, *"We concluded that for patients with low back pain, treatment with TENS is no more effective than treatment with a placebo."*[6]

Microcurrent therapy (MENS) is a new form of electrotherapy which claims to produce "outstanding pain relief and accelerated healing."[14] MENS uses an electrical current of small amperage (10-600 microamps) at a level below that of sensory perception; it is thought to stimulate healing in body tissues.

Traction

Traction is a form of mobilization in which an outside force is used to elongate the spine. The amount of pull and position of the patient can vary; traditionally the patient is backlying with about 20 pounds of pull applied from a pelvic belt. For neck pain, traction is applied in sitting with a chin harness. Also used are higher amounts of pressure, prone traction and gravity traction, (where the patient is suspended from a ribcage harness or hangs upside down with gravity boots). While some practitioners use 18-25 pounds of traction constantly for weeks at a time, others use 80-200 pounds daily for one-half hour for up to two weeks. There is some indication that the heavier traction, when used for appropriate symptoms, is more effective.[3] [See Box 4-2]

Effects of Traction

- separation of vertebral bodies and facet joints
- tensing of ligaments
- straightening of spinal curves
- stiffening of the annular fibers of the disks to minimize bulging of the nucleus
- decreasing tension on nerve roots and dura (covering of the nerve root)
- realigning vertebrae to relive a nerve root compression
- stretching spinal muscles to reduce spasm.

The degree of flexion or extension in positioning the patient determines which of these is the most pronounced.

Box 4-2

The benefits of traction are controversial; some physicians never recommend it.[7] Traction may increase pain because additional fluid is absorbed by the nucleus of the disk during the procedure; disk pressure is then increased when the traction is released.

Manual traction is used by some practitioners during spinal manipulation; this is covered in Chapter 12, "Manual Therapy."

Mechanical Supports

Mechanical supports can immobilize a body part or correct poor alignment; they come in many forms, such as braces, corsets, cervical collars, casts, shoe inserts and traction slings. [See Box 4-3]

Supports are prescribed to produce one of the following effects:
- immobilization
- increased movement of adjacent segments
- transfer of weight and movement away from the spine to other structures
- increased abdominal support
- decreased pressure on the disks
- assistance in venous return (blood flow to the heart)
- control of lumbar lordosis or thoracic kyphosis
- increased patient awareness of correct posture
- decreased use of spinal muscles for relief of spasm
- a placebo effect where the use of a support gives the patient a sense of security

Box 4-3

Rigid braces and casts are inappropriate for many back pain patients, because the goal in treatment is to promote normal movement of the spine. An "Elasticon" garment is preferred by some practitioners due to its considerable comfort and its usefulness in both providing support and allowing almost full spinal movement during treatment.[9] Because the spine has a different configuration in different positions, a support does not fit well in all positions; it must be customized for each individual.

The sacro-iliac joint is an area with essentially no muscular support; with chronic sacro-iliac joint dysfunction a sacral support may be necessary. A belt which surrounds the pelvis at hip level with a stabilization pad over the sacrum is used. The combination of forces created on the sacrum, pelvis and soft tissues of the region by the pad and belt, stabilize the joint while still allowing lumbar movement.[2,15]

Supports may increase comfort but they don't speed healing. Braces, corsets and cervical collars should be used as a short-term solution; they should never be prescribed without a plan to eliminate them.[8,15] Total dependency on a brace allows the soft tissues of the spine to relinquish their supporting function so that the brace becomes the sole support. It should be fully explained to the patient that a mechanical support is a temporary measure and an exercise/posture/body mechanics program should be initiated simultaneously.[5]

Equipment

Recovering from back pain often requires relearning proper posture and body mechanics. Prescription and non-prescription equipment is available to help patients maintain a proper position. Sitting is often difficult, especially for those with disk problems. [See Box 4-4]

Examples of Seating Supports

- An "ergonomic chair" is fully adjustable; it promotes a posture of knees at 90 degrees of flexion, trunk at 10-20 degrees back from vertical and the lumbar curve supported four inches from the seat.[13]
- The Balans Multi-Chair, (with a forward sloping seat, knee pads and no back support), puts the user's weight onto the knees; this encourages maintenance of lumbar lordosis and spinal muscle activity more effectively than straight back or office chairs.
- Molded car seats maintain and support the lumbar curve; riding in a car is especially harmful for disk patients due to the flexed position and high frequency vibrations.
- A wedge can turn a back sloping seat into a more upright one; this is helpful in preventing slouch sitting.
- Other commercially available chairs which are adjustable or provide more forward tilting back support are the "Pos" chair, "Inclination stool" and the "Pendulum."[10]

See Chapter 8, "Posture and Body Mechanics," for specific recommendations concerning proper postures in sitting.

Box 4-4

A variety of positioning and exercise equipment which is available to the general public comes with grandiose claims about health benefits.

"Many users have found that Nordic Track relieves back pain." (skiing treadmill)

"Reduce or eliminate low back pain! . . . an excellent remedy for the back pain patient who truly wants to get back to a normal pain-free lifestyle" (seated lumbar traction)

"No more neck aches" (sleep pillow)
"Help prevent and relieve pain and stiffness." (cervical pillow)
"Probably the most effective aid yet produced for back pain relief while sitting" (seat cushion)
"Say goodby to your chronic nagging backache." (seat cushion)

Exercise equipment, such as the Nordic Track and stair climbing machines, are meant to strengthen back muscles. Gravity boots, gravity tables and "The Orthopod" provide traction to the spine. Needless to say, equipment which is advertised as the cure for back pain is suspect. Consumers should objectively determine an item's purpose and decide if it can address their specific dysfunctions. This is the only way to decide if a piece of equipment can have a useful role in an overall, individualized rehabilitation program.

Massage, medications, relaxation techniques, exercise and posture/body mechanics programs may all be recommended in a conservative approach to back pain. These will be discussed in depth in later chapters.

Key Points - Conservative Treatment

The majority of patients with back pain are advised to try conservative measures before extensive diagnostic testing or invasive procedures are initiated. The treatments discussed in this section include bedrest, physical agents, traction, mechanical supports and equipment for seating and exercise. They are not effective in curing back pain, but can provide temporary, symptomatic relief and be used to assist active movement. However, their overuse can be more detrimental than the original problem; prolonged or total bedrest, for example, is now recognized to cause both physical and psychological harm and in most cases is not necessary.

Footnotes

1 "Approaches to Musculoskeletal Problems: Focus on the Low Back" Symposium, Stephen McDavitt
2 *The Back Letter*, Vol. 4, No. 2
3 Ben Benjamin, "The Mystery of Lower Back Pain"

4   Rene Cailliet, *Low Back Pain Syndrome*, 1962 edition
5   Rene Cailliet, *Low Back Pain Syndrome*, 1988 edition
6   Richard Deyo, et al., "A Controlled Trial of Transcutaneous Electrical Nerve
    Stimulation (TENS) and Exercise for Chronic Low Back Pain"
7   Charles Fager, "Beware the Quick Fix for Back Pain"
8   Kaplan & Tanner, *Musculoskelatal Pain and Disability*
9   W.H. Kirkaldy-Willis, *Managing Back Pain*
10 Steve Marantz, "The Perfect Chair"
11 James McGavin, "The McKenzie Approach to Spinal Pain"
12 David Miller, "Comparison of Electromyographic Activity in the Lumbar
    Paraspinal Muscles of Subjects with and without Low Back Pain"
13 Paulette Olsen, "Brief Media Presentation on Back Care"
14 Robert Picker, "Microcurrent Therapy: 'Jump-Starting Healing with Bioelectricity'"
15 Duane Saunders, *Evaluation, Treatment and Prevention of Musculoskeletal
    Disorders*
16 Richard Sternbach, *Pain Patients: Traits and Treatments*

Chapter 5 - Medications

"The desire to take medicine is perhaps the greatest feature which distinguishes man from animals." Sir William Osler

The medications which are used for people with back pain may be prescribed to inhibit pain, decrease inflammation, relax muscles, decrease tension or elevate mood. They include the following:

- NSAIDs (non-steroidal anti-inflammatory drugs) - decrease pain and inflammation [see Box 5-1]
- aspirin (salicylates) - decrease pain and inflammation
- opiates - decrease pain
- barbituates - decrease pain
- tranquilizers - decrease emotional tension [see Box 5-1]
- antidepressants - elevate mood [see Box 5-1]
- muscle relaxants - decrease muscle tension [see Box 5-1]

NSAIDs, Valium and Anti-Depressants

NSAIDs are routinely prescribed for soft tissue injuries for weeks or even months; they are thought to contribute to a quicker and better recovery, but research does not uniformly support such an assumption.[1] After an acute injury, inflammation may be excessive and NSAIDs can help to reduce it. However, inflammation is a normal response of the body and probably shouldn't be obliterated.[1] With ongoing back pain the rationale for using NSAIDs is questionable because the cause of the pain may not involve inflammation.

Valium is often prescribed for pain, due to its properties as a muscle relaxant and tranquilizer. However, the drug seems to increase the subjective pain experience and increase feelings of confusion and helplessness;[2] it is now known to have addictive potential with heavy long-term use.

There has recently been success in the use of **anti-depressants** for chronic pain. In one study, patients taking the anti-depressant "amitripyline" became more active with less pain; a comparison group received psychotherapy and, although more productive, reported more pain.[1]

Box 5-1

Certain medications can be helpful during acute episodes and others appropriate for people with chronic pain. However, back pain patients are advised to minimize drug use to avoid the dangers of side effects and physical or emotional addiction. Drug abuse is one of the most devastating complications with chronic pain. Patients can become addicted to pain-killing or other medications; they may even use the pain to justify continued drug use instead or taking more positive measures.[2]

Holistic health practitioners have even stronger objections to the use of medications than the fear of addiction. They believe that synthesized chemicals cannot possibly promote healing or sustain health.[3] Chemical treatments, including antibiotics and immunizations, are thought to meddle with the immune system and interfere with self-healing, causing rather than curing serious health problems.[3]

Key Points - Medications

There are a variety of prescription medications for back pain patients which may be helpful for acute or chronic pain. However, drug use carries with it the risk of side effects and physical or emotional addiction. Medications usually treat the symptoms of back pain, not the causes, and their use should be minimized.

Footnotes

1 *The Back Letter,* Vol. 4, No. 6
2 Steven Brena, *Chronic Pain: America's Hidden Epidemic*
3 Annemarie Colbin, *Food and Healing*

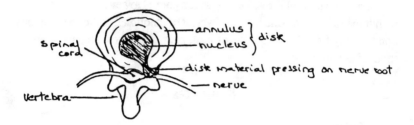

Figure 6-1. Vertebra, top view, with a ruptured disk compressing a nerve root.

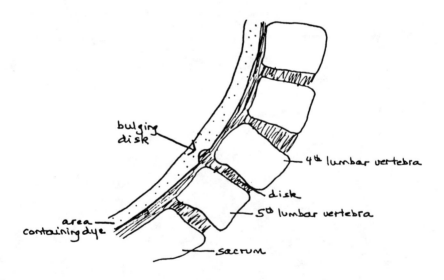

Figure 6-2. Representation of a myelogram showing a prolapsed disk between the fourth and fifth lumbar vertebrae which may or may not be causing pain.

Chapter 6 - Surgery

"70-80 percent of patients with low back pain who are screened carefully for radicular symptoms benefit from surgery." Rene Cailliet, MD[2]

"Surgery fails completely in 20 percent of patients with low back pain and 60 percent continue to have symptoms." David Imrie, MD[5]

People often believe that surgery is performed when other treatments fail - that it is the drastic but sure answer which will relieve their symptoms. In fact, surgery does not help most back pain patients. In one study, the advantage of surgery over conservative treatment, based on improved function and decreased symptoms, was not statistically significant after 4 or 10 years.[9] It is estimated that, at most, 10 percent of the patients with low back pain have disk problems and only 1 percent have true disk ruptures, which is one of the few indications for an operation.[2] That means that well over 90 percent of those with back problems cannot be helped by surgery.[1]

Approximately 200,000 operations/year are done in the U.S. to remove the ruptured nucleus of a disk;[12] this procedure is called a "diskectomy." Up to 40 percent of these are "failed back surgeries";[2] the failure is often in the interpretation of the findings which led to surgical intervention.[4] Surgery should be reserved for patients with unmistakable evidence of nerve root compression, [see Figure 6-1], or cauda equina syndrome, [see Box 6-1]. Too many operations are performed due to misinterpreted radiographic findings; the bulging disks seen on CAT scans and MRIs are common and often asymptomatic.[4] X-rays cannot visualize disks at all; CAT scans, MRI, diskography, thermography and EMG are not reliable disk diagnosers. Even myelography has false positives and negatives. [See Figure 6-2] All diagnostic testing should be used to confirm what is already suspected from the history and physical exam.[2]

Cauda Equina Syndrome

The cauda equina syndrome, characterized by bladder symptoms, is the exception to a conservative approach to operating. Nerve compression from a disk rupture which affects sacral nerves can result in loss of bladder emptying tone, of bladder capacity sensation and of sphincter function. Relieving the compression is urgent; if this condition is not treated promptly, permanent bladder dysfunction can result.

Box 6-1

Referral to a surgeon is appropriate when a patient has the following symptoms:[4]
- unremitting radiating pain
- the presence of neurologic signs (numbness, weakness, decreased reflexes)
- incapacitating or intolerable pain
- bowel or bladder symptoms
- significant or suddenly progressive muscle weakness.

Most patients with disk problems improve without surgery so that conservative treatment is recommended for 4-6 weeks. If symptoms do not subside after this time, radiographic studies are then indicated. Since the primary role of surgery is to relieve nerve root compression, bony fusion of vertebrae is not always necessary following disk removal. In a fusion, chips of bone from another part of the patient's body are placed between the vertebrae, immobilizing that segment as they grow together. Fusions are now done less frequently and the recurrence rate of symptoms is similar with and without fusion.[4] Disk herniations from a traumatic injury and the simultaneous rupture of two or more disks are unusual, therefore it is rare that removal of more than one disk is required.

In addition to ruptured disks, another source of nerve root compression and pain is bone spurs. These are common and asymptomatic in many people, but if they are pushing against a spinal nerve they can cause severe symptoms.

Even with a successful surgical procedure, failed back surgery can result due to post-operative adhesions, scarring or nerve root adherence. Follow-up therapy is important, (such as passive straight leg raising every two hours immediately post-op), for optimum results. Even when surgery is indicated and provides dramatic relief of symptoms, it does not correct the underlying disorder which led to the nerve root compression.

Alternative Surgery for Disk Rupture

A number of alternative procedures have been touted for less invasive pain-relief than a diskectomy; these remain controversial. Some surgeons feel that they offer no advantages over traditional surgery, may necessitate further procedures, fail to relieve symptoms or can be harmful.[4]

Microsurgery, Suction and Chemonucleolysis

1) Microsurgery is said to be less costly and less traumatic than diskectomy. It uses magnification of the operating field and thereby requires a smaller incision with less scarring and shorter hospitalization.

2) "Percutaneous automated discectomy" uses suction to remove the extruded fragment of the damaged disk and boasts fewer risks of complication than with traditional surgery.

3) Injection of the enzyme "chymopapain" from the papaya plant provides a nonsurgical approach through "chemonucleolysis" (chemical destruction of the nucleus of the disk through enzyme action). Although there are claims that half of the people needing disk surgery could benefit from chymopapain injection,[11] it seems to be least effective for complete ruptures, i.e., for the patients who most need surgery.[4] In addition, one percent of patients have life-threatening allergic reactions to the enzyme. Chymopapain can also cause severe neurological damage if it leaks into cerebro-spinal fluid; it can destroy healthy tissue if injected into the outer disk versus the extruded fragment, and may speed disk degeneration.[4]

Surgery can be a dramatically successful approach to back pain, but the key is limiting it to appropriate patients with specific pathology. Patients who shop around until they find a surgeon willing to operate have a very good chance of increasing their disability and their pain.

Invasive Procedures for Chronic Pain

Surgery or injection is occasionally used for patients with severe chronic pain which has not responded to other treatments. The procedure in these cases is not to relieve nerve root compression, but to block pain.

1) "Neuroaugmentive" surgery is done for patients with symptoms of chronic dull, aching pain. A device is implanted under the skin; it provides electronic stimulation which blocks the transmission of pain messages.

2) "Deafferation," (such as rhizotomy, cordotomy, dorsal root entry zone radiofrequency lesions or intracranial procedures), controls pain by severing or destroying a sensory nerve. In facet rhizotomy or radiofrequency facet denervation, the sensory nerves around the facet joint are cut or burned in order to provide pain relief. Critics of these procedures state that the nerve supply to other structures, (e.g. ligaments and the small spinal muscles), is also affected; this may contribute to further facet joint instability and trauma.[7,8]

3) Patients with pain due to nerve root compression can receive a steroid injection into the space surrounding the spinal cord and nerve roots; this treatment is called an epidural injection. It decreases pain without significantly interfering with sensory or motor nerves. Advocates of epidural injections claim it provides immediate pain relief in 80 percent of patients;[10] the effects gradually dissolve over the following six months. One study, however, found no difference in pain relief between patients receiving an epidural injection and those who were injected with a placebo.[3] One risk of epidural injection is incorrect placement of the needle, which happens up to 25 percent of the time;[10] serious complications include infections or inflammation of the meninges (the three outer coverings of the brain and spinal cord).[3]

4) Injection of a pain-killing substance with or without steroids can be used for diagnostic or therapeutic purposes in spinal or pelvic structures. If anesthetizing a facet joint provides dramatic relief, it identifies

the site of the pain and may justify more extreme measures. The effects of a steroid injection may last months. However, over time repeated injections can destroy soft tissue.

5) "Proliferant" injections are sometimes used when pain results from sprained or stretched ligaments; the purpose is to stimulate the production of new tissue to strengthen the ligaments. Repeated injection therapy over one to two months is usually necessary.

6) Manipulation under anesthesia is used at one hospital which claims a success rate of 25 percent cured, 50 percent much improved, and 20 percent better.[6] The program incorporates a wide variety of traditional and alternative approaches into a treatment regime. These are followed by vigorous manipulation of hypomobile joints, which is performed with the patient anesthetized.[6]

Key Points - Surgery

Although surgery is assumed by many to be the ultimate cure when other treatments fail, it is in fact inappropriate for the majority of back pain patients. There are very specific conditions under which referral to a surgeon is appropriate, specifically symptoms of nerve root compression which have not responded to conservative treatment. There are several new surgical procedures for ruptured disks, but traditional "diskectomy" remains the treatment of choice. There are also surgical procedures for chronic pain patients; these are done to block pain, but may provide only temporary relief.

Chapter 6

Footnotes

1 Edward Abraham, *Freedom from Back Pain*
2 Rene Cailliet, *Low Back Pain Syndrome*
3 John Cuckler, et al., "The Use of Epidural Steroids in the Treatment of Lumbar Radicular Pain"
4 Charles Fager, "The Neurosurgical Management of Lumbar Spine Disease"
5 David Imrie, *Goodbye Back Ache*
6 Krumhansl & Nowacek, "Case Study - Spinal Manipulation Under Anaesthesia"
7 Stanley Paris, "Anatomy as Related to Functional Pain"
8 Stanley Paris, "Physical Signs of Instability"
9 Jo Solet, "Low Back Pain - An Overview"
10 Arthur White, "Injection Techniques for the Diagnosis and Treatment of Low Back Pain"
11 Judith Willis, "Back Pain: Ubiquitous, Controversial"
12 David Zinman, "Focus on Back Pain"

Chapter 7 - Relaxation Techniques

"Warning: Aggravation Ahead" Highway Department Sign on Rte. 270 entering Washington D.C.

Rehabilitation for a back problem incorporates increased activity alternated with relaxation in order to diminish pain and allow healing. Relaxation techniques may be used to reduce muscle spasm or stretch tight muscles. Other types of relaxation training reduce anxiety and improve a patient's sense of control; patients are encouraged to gain mental mastery over their tension. Many programs emphasize the importance of combining physical and mental relaxation. A partial list of the numerous methods used to promote relaxation follows:

- exercises+
- physical conditioning+

- progressive relaxation exercises (including Jacobson's)
- Alexander Technique*
- dance therapy+
- breathing exercises (including Fuch's and Jenck's)
- acupuncture and acupressure*
- counseling
- meditation
- meditation on a single word or color (Benson's Technique or The Relaxation Response)
- behavior modification (receiving a reward for a desired physical response)
- energetics (combining body movements and verbalizations for the release of blocked enery and reintegration of mind and body)
- mental training exercises such as autogenic training (mental focusing on a short verbal phrase which suggests a state of physiological balance - "My arms and legs are warm." "My heartbeat is calm and regular.")
- visualization*
- hypnosis or self-hypnosis
- biofeedback
- muscle inhibition techniques (including reciprocal inhibition, muscle fatigue and strain-counterstrain)
- disciplines for mind and body (including yoga, Tai Chi and Zen)
- massage

+ These treatment approaches are discussed in other chapters in PART 1.
* These treatment approaches are discussed in PART 2.

Hypnosis, Biofeedback and Muscle Inhibition

Hypnosis is guided, altered attention; the focus is on the power of the mind to solve a specific problem. The patient's concept of what is happening changes, for example feelings of panic subside; then the body responds to what the mind perceives. For back pain patients, the mind is guided to overcome fear, pain or any perceived mechanical limitation which influences the body.[2] Hypnosis can be used for relaxation and to widen a patient's focus. However, it is not very effective for chronic pain patients when environmental factors are reinforcing the pain behavior.[1]

In **biofeedback**, patients have electrodes attached to skin surfaces; these are connected to a machine which monitors muscle contractions. The activity of spastic or tense muscles is visually presented on the machine, or represented by auditory signals. From seeing or hearing this feedback, patients can learn to consciously relax their muscles.

Physical therapists try to use the patient's own nervous system to relax or stretch tight muscles. In one **muscle inhibition** technique, the therapist passively lengthens a muscle immediately following a strong, resisted contraction; the contraction is automatically followed by relaxation of the muscle through nervous system mechanisms. Having the assistance of the nervous system is both more effective and less painful than forcing a muscle to stretch.

Yoga and Tai Chi

Yoga is an Eastern mind-body approach that promotes relaxation, flexibility and strength, as well as mental discipline. It uses positive mental suggestions with breathing patterns, body and mind moving together. The energy flow generated is thought to promote physical fitness and mental well-being. Postures ("asanas") for the back include cobra (press-up), locust (prone with the lower body lifted in hyperextension) and neck roll and twist. Yoga claims benefits specifically for back pain patients. It is one of the more successful treatments for the prevention of back problems or for alleviating minor back pain.[5] Yoga teachers with expertise in backs are often able to tailor an exercise program to meet the back pain patient's needs. Yoga, however, may be too strenuous for certain back conditions.

Tai Chi is another ancient Chinese system of exercise which promotes relaxation; it is said to offer a mental and physical outlet and to produce effects similar to meditation. Tai Chi consists of exercises carried out in a continuous, non-strenuous manner. All parts of the body are exercised, enhancing flexibility, strength, cardiovascular fitness, coordination and good posture.

Massage

Massage is the treatment most often associated with relaxation. For those with or without serious health problems, it can relieve physical and emotional tension. It is usually performed by physical therapists or massage therapists and comes in many forms. With back pain, massage is used to decrease muscle spasm, increase circulation, free adhesions, decrease pain sensitivity and reduce scar tissue; together these effects are thought to speed the healing process. Massage often follows heat or cold treatment and is done in a relaxing rhythm. It should be deep enough to gradually restore tissue to its normal, soft, elongated, nontender state.[4] [See Box 7-1]

Friction Massage

Deep friction massage is done directly to an injured site; the therapist's fingers and patient's skin move together in a direction perpendicular to the normal orientation of the muscle fibers. It is done to increase stretchability and mobility with chronic lesions of soft tissue. It helps maintain mobility with respect to adjacent tissues, but without stressing the injured fibers in the longitudinal direction. Deep friction massage is also thought to promote the normal orientation of new fibers as they're produced.[3,4]

Box 7-1

There is little evidence that massage alone can eliminate back pain, other than making patients feel better temporarily.[4] It is an appropriate therapeutic tool when it can actually reduce tissue pathology; this includes (1) decreasing muscle tension which is perpetuating the pathology, (2) increasing stretchability of fibers, (3) increasing circulation and (4) increasing mobility between tissue surfaces.[4] [See Box 7-2]

Indications for Massage
- ischemia (decreased circulation)
- scarring or adhesions
- edema (tissue swelling)
- muscle spasm or tension
- poor tissue nutrition
- trigger points (tender, fibrous areas in muscles)
- emotional stress

Any of these factors may be associated with pain.

Indications for Friction Massage

Injuries involving . . .

muscles - recent trauma with inflammation, long-standing scars or lesions at the muscle-tendon juncture

tendons - tenosynovitis, tendonitis

ligaments - recent or chronic sprain

Box 7-2

The American Massage Therapy Association recommends that students in schools for massage receive a minimum of 500 hours of classroom instruction. The curriculum includes basic sciences (anatomy, physiology, kinesiology), massage theory and practical work. MTs currently become certified by becoming active members of their national organization upon graduation.

Key Points - Relaxation Techniques

There are a large number of relaxation techniques available to decrease muscle spasm, emotional tension or both. The most well-known, massage, is useful for people with back pain under the following circumstances:
- to reduce muscular and emotional tension
- to increase circulation and reduce swelling
- to free adhesions and restore tissue mobility.

Used alone, relaxation techniques do not usually produce dramatic long-term relief for back problems.

Footnotes

1 "Approaches to Musculoskeletal Problems: Focus on the Low Back" Symposium, Jane Derebery
2 Sarah Carroll, "Hypnosis: An Underutilized Modality"
3 James Cyriax, *Textbook of Orthopaedic Medicine*
4 Kessler & Hertling, *Management of Common Musculoskeletal Disorders*
5 Klein & Sobel, *Backache Relief*

Chapter 8 - Posture and Body Mechanics

"The spine is poorly designed for standing erect." Philip Gildenberg & Richard DeVaul[2]
"Back problems are often due to excessive sitting in our society." James McGavin, PT[5]
"If you have chronic low back pain, the blame probably lies with the way you use your back." Deborah Caplan[1]

Posture is the position one assumes against gravity; body mechanics is the posture of the body in motion. The goal of good posture is to maintain balanced alignment against gravity with the minimum use of energy. The spine has four continuous curves for flexibility and shock absorption; energy efficient posture requires that the normal curves are maintained to put the muscles at optimum working length. [See Figure 8-1] The spinal column is supported by a complex system of muscles, ligaments and joints, all working together. Ligamentous support occurs without energy expenditure; muscle action intervenes at the limits of ligament stress. Poor posture causes reduced efficiency in the skeletal/ligament systems; a prolonged position of poor

77

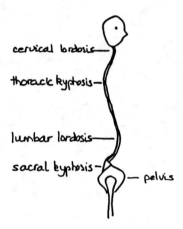

Figure 8-1. Correct standing posture, side view, characterized by the maintenance of the natural curves of the spine.

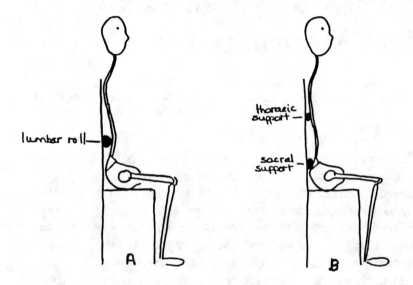

Figure 8-2. (A) Use of a lumbar roll in sitting to maintain a lumbar lordosis. (B) Use of a thoracic and sacral support for spinal stability in sitting.

posture, with flattened or exaggerated curves, overstretches and overworks the muscles. For example, the neck supports the weight of the head, normally 8-12 pounds. When an individual sits with the head hanging forward, a torque is created at the base of the neck, increasing the force of the head on the neck to as much as 36 pounds.[7]

As people grow older, changes occur which are probably due more to lifestyle than physiological aging. The muscles lose tone and become deconditioned. The head juts forward, shoulders sag, chest sinks, butt and abdomen protrude and the spine curves. Flexibility and range of motion are lost; muscles, tendons and ligaments shorten. With an increasingly slouched posture, added stress is put on muscles and spinal structures, so that vertebrae and disks are pulled out of their normal alignment. The whole spinal structure becomes weakened and more vulnerable to injury. When pain is suddenly elicited during a specific incident, the assumption is often made that something has slipped our of place or snapped. Most back and neck problems, however, are probably not caused by a single injury; a healthy back is unlikely to be hurt by a single twist, lift or fall.[8] Much more commonly, symptoms are the result of months or years of stress to the spine from poor posture, faulty body mechanics, stressful working and living habits, loss of flexibility and general decline of physical fitness.[6]

Poor posture is a possible cause of or contributing factor toward dysfunction in any spinal structure. Proper posture and body mechanics is one of the few treatment approaches which is advised for virtually every person with back pain, as well as for prevention. No treatment can undo the harmful effects of continual misuse of the back, but it is never too late to learn how to stand, sit, bend, lift and sleep correctly.

Treatment to Improve Posture and Body Mechanics

"Good posture hinges on the pelvic tilt." David Imrie, MD[3] / *"Avoid swayback at all times."* William Ishmael, MD, & Howard Shorbe, MD[4]

"The usual recommendation to pelvic tilt is bad for the spine as it prevents free use of the hip joint, increasing strain on the lower back, and keeps the spine from efficient vertical alignment." Deborah Caplan[1]

Adjusting the body's posture and movement, unlike treatments such as manipulation or surgery, is one of the few approaches which is universally helpful for every back pain patient. Unfortunately, treatment is often limited to the acutely painful phase of an episode with no follow-up to optimize strength, flexibility and posture. Part of a rehabilitation program should include an individualized assessment of a patient's posture and body mechanics. Many Physical Therapy departments offer "Back School," a class to teach proper use of the back. Patients then need to make these new habits permanent.

For many years, flattening the lumbar lordosis through the "pelvic tilt routine" was considered the appropriate approach for protecting the back. Most specialists now recommend maintenance of the natural, gentle curves of neck and back during all activities. A degree of lordosis is encouraged as desirable and physiologically sound. Flattening or bowing out the lower back overstretches soft tissues and increases pressure on the disks. Excessive lordosis also stresses the back, especially those structures at the apex of the curve. These effects are exaggerated by obesity which further increases the curve and adds wear and tear on the joints and disks; part of a posture program includes the recommendation for weight loss, if appropriate.

It is difficult to remain comfortable in one position for more than an hour. Whatever the activity, (sitting, driving, lying down, etc.), changing position frequently is recommended in order to unload joints, relax muscles and redistribute pressure on weight-bearing surfaces.

Specific Recommendations for Posture

Sitting

Prolonged sitting is a stressful position for the spine; sitting for even brief periods can be difficult for those with disk problems.

- Sit so that your knees are at about the same level as your hips.
- Sit as close to your work surface as possible.
- Avoid sitting for long periods without getting up, walking around and stretching into extension.
- In the office, your desk should be at elbow height or higher and chairs should be adjustable.
- Add supports to your chair to increase spinal stability and comfort. A lumbar roll is placed at waist level to maintain a lordosis for those with disk problems. Sacral and thoracic support may be more comfortable for some. [See Figure 8-2]

- Use arm rests to further reduce the load on your back.
- A recommended back height for chairs is from four inches above the seat to just below the shoulder blades, with the back about 10-20 degrees from vertical. (See "Equipment for Positioning" in Chapter 4, for specific chair designs.)

Driving

- Driving requires good support for the lower back. Riding in a car stresses the disks while simultaneously fatiguing the muscles; the vibrations of travel make it hard for the muscles to work effectively.
- Your trunk should be about 10-20 degrees from vertical; a wedge-shaped back support can be used to achieve a comfortable angle.
- A lumbar roll can be used to support your lumbar spine and maintain a lordosis; thoracic and sacral supports can be used to stabilize the spine. [See Figure 8-2]
- The seat should be moved forward or a seat cushion used so that your knees are at about the same height as the seat.
- On long drives, try to stop periodically to stand up, walk around and stretch into extension.
- Avoid strenuous motions when first getting out of a car to allow your back time to recover from prolonged sitting.
- Immediately after driving, stretch back into extension and avoid bending and lifting for about 10 minutes.

Standing

- If standing for long periods, change position often, putting alternate feet up on a low support.
- Have work at a comfortable height so you don't have to lean forward to reach it.
- Wear comfortable shoes, not very high heels or platforms that jeopardize balance.

Lifting

Many back problems result (or are aggravated) from lifting improperly; they are most apt to occur with sudden jerking and twisting movements. The standard recommendation for lifting used to be to keep

the lower back flattened and lean forward when rising. However, it is now recognized that this position can overstretch soft tissues and increase pressure on the disks. [See Figure 8-3]
- Maintain a lumbar lordosis while lifting.
- Avoid twisting and bending or twisting while rising.
- For a diagonal lift, keep the object in front of you with one foot in front of your body and one behind to give a wide balanced base of support.
- Use the muscles of your legs and buttocks to rise while your abdominals and back extensors stabilize your spine; keep the object as close to your body as possible.
- If possible, use your arms to help push up to standing. Move your feet to turn, rather than twisting your trunk.
- Carry loads at your sides or on your shoulders rather than in front, preferably with equal weights on left and right sides.
- When an object is too heavy to lift or carry, get help.
- Above all, determine whether it is necessary or appropriate for you to be lifting this particular object.

Lying down
- Sleep on a mattress that is firm, but can conform to your body's normal curves; waterbeds are satisfactory if adequately filled.
- Change position periodically while resting to reduce stress on your joints and muscles.
- Find the position most comfortable for you so that you can truly rest.
- Use a pillow that supports your neck, so that it is resting in a balanced position with a normal lordosis.
- Sleeping on your stomach is not necessarily bad with a firm mattress; this may be a comfortable position for those with disk problems.
- In backlying, a balanced position can be promoted with a small pillow under your knees.
- In sidelying, put a pillow between your legs with your lower leg nearly straight and your top leg bent.
- In stomachlying, don't use a pillow for your head but try one under your lower shins for increased comfort.

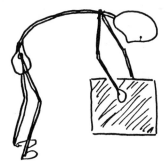

Figure 8-3. Lifting with a flattened lumbar spine which increases stress on the disks.

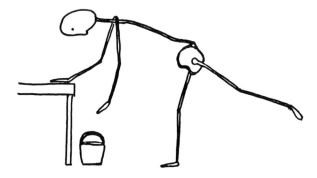

Figure 8-4. Golfer's lift which maintains the natural curves of the spine during forward bending.

Specific Recommendations for Body Mechanics

- Maintain the balanced position for your back (with natural curves) for all activities.
- Use your arms for support in moving from one position to another.
- Minimize twisting and bending at the same time.
- Tighten your stomach muscles in preparation for lifting or changing position.
- Get close to the activity you're involved in to minimize excessive reaching, slouching or lunging to a new position.
- Avoid quick, jerky movements.
- Change position frequently when working at one task.
- To avoid excessive sitting, try performing activities in kneeling or on all fours.
- For dressing and foot care, keep one leg extended while flexing the other to reach your foot; avoid pants or footwear that are a struggle to put on.
- During acutely painful episodes when prolonged sitting on the toilet is necessary, face backwards and lean on the tank for support.
- Use a lumbar roll, thoracic or sacral supports for activities involving prolonged sitting.
- Change position or split up tasks into enough steps to avoid unbalanced transitions or excessive strain.
- Use the "golfer's lift," with one leg extended, when bending forward from standing. [See Figure 8-4]
- Find positions for sexual activity which are not stressful to the spine.
- Ask for help when necessary.
- Ask yourself if it's really necessary to do this activity.
- Pace yourself and break up difficult tasks with rest periods.

There are excellent guides for posture and body mechanics for people with all levels of back pain. Many are inexpensive and well worth reading and applying so that the spine won't continue to be subjected to repeated injury and stress through improper use. *Managing Back Pain, For Your*

Neck, Sex and Back Pain and other booklets are available from Educational Opportunities in Bloomington, Minnesota; call 1-800-654-8357 for a catalog.

Key Points - Posture and Body Mechanics

Using proper posture and body mechanics is recommended for everybody - for minimizing back pain, preventing its occurrence or reoccurrence and for giving other treatment approaches the best chance for success. The postural changes associated with aging weaken the entire spinal structure and make the back more vulnerable to injury; years of preventable abuse may cause many back and neck problems. General rules for reducing spinal stress include maintenance of the natural curves of the back and changing position frequently. Specific recommendations are detailed in this chapter.

Footnotes

1 Deborah Caplan, *Back Trouble*
2 Gildenberg & DeVaul, *The Chronic Pain Patient*
3 David Imrie, *Goodbye Back Ache*
4 Ishmael & Shorbe, "Care of the Back"
5 James McGavin, "The McKenzie Approach to Spinal Pain"
6 Melnick, et al., *Managing Back Pain*
7 Paulette Olsen, "Brief Media Presentation on Back Care"
8 Duane Saunders, *The Back Care Program*

Chapter 9 - Back Exercises

"The best ultimate therapy is an exercise program to strengthen muscles of the region."
Charles Fager, MD[7]
"Exercise routines have no place in the treatment of spinal dysfunction." Stanley Paris,
PT[13]

Physical conditioning seems to benefit all kinds of back problems, but there is insufficient information regarding the effects of specific exercises on back pain. No support exists for the use of preprinted handouts which assumes every patient with back pain requires the same exercise routine; specific exercises should be selected on the basis of a thorough physical evaluation.

Exercises may be prescribed for back pain patients to (1) regain or acquire adequate flexibility of soft tissues and/or (2) regain or acquire adequate strength of the muscles related to back function.

Flexibility Exercises - With full movement and no pain at the end of range of motion, it is probably not necessary to work on flexibility of that motion; it is possible to be too flexible, overstretching and weakening joints and muscles. When stretching a muscle, a sustained position of stretch is vastly preferable to a quick stretch or to "bouncing"; these physiologically encourage the muscle to fight the stretch. All range of motion exercises should be done slowly for both protection of tissues and maximum effectiveness. Methods that inhibit a muscle by using the body's own nervous system mechanisms are the most effective and comfortable techniques for lengthening a tight muscle; (this concept was discussed in Chapter 7 under "Muscle Inhibition").

Strengthening Exercises - Strengthening exercises should address opposing muscle groups so that balanced muscle strength is achieved. Muscles must become fatigued for exercises to be most effective; as a weak muscle grows stronger, more repetition or resistance is added to continue improvement. Generally, high resistance exercises build strength while repetitive exercises build endurance. Exercises should be performed slowly and done consistently, (4-7 times/week). Exercises that increase pain are probably contraindicated, while those that reduce pain are probably beneficial, contradicting the "no pain, no gain" philosophy.[6] [See Box 9-1]

Types of Movement and Muscle Action

1) **Active** movement - A muscle contracts in response to nerve (or electrical) stimulation; this is the only way to strengthen a muscle.

2) **Passive** movement - A body part is moved by an outside force; this mobilizes the joint but has no effect on muscle strength and burns no calories.

3) **Resisted** movement - A muscle actively works against resistance from an outside force or a mechanical object such as a weight; this builds maximum strength. Resistance can be given throughout the range of motion or can be so strong that no movement is permitted.

4) **Shortening** contraction - The muscle actively contracts, shortening to move a body part; this is the most traditional way to exercise muscles.

5) **Isometric** contraction - The muscle tenses, but no movement results. Isometrics are useful for acutely painful episodes when repetitive movement would be too stressful on spinal structures. They can also be done against strong resistance to build holding power.

6) **Lengthening** contraction - A motion is reversed with a controlled, slow return to the starting position, with or without resistance. Lengthening contractions are thought to be at least as efficient in building strength as shortening contractions.

Gravity is a significant factor in exercise; it can either assist or resist a movement and determines which muscles are being exercised. For example, slowly straightening the knee in sitting exercises the knee *extensor* muscles; slowly straightening the knee in prone (stomachlying) exercises the knee *flexor* muscles. In the first, gravity resists knee extension and in the second assists it; in prone, the knee flexor muscles have to work to control the lowering of the leg.

Box 9-1

Chapter 9

Flexion Exercises

For a long time, flexion was considered the answer for back pain, and flexion routines were prescribed for all patients. "Williams flexion exercises" (pelvic tilts, gluteal sets, knee to chest, sit-ups) were first developed in 1937 and have long been the mainstay for low back problems. Flexion flattens the lumbar curve of the spine, separates the facet joints and stretches back extensors. Strong trunk flexor muscles (the abdominals) have long been thought to reduce stress on spinal structures. Not everyone, however, agrees on the role of flexion in reducing back pain.

"A low back is as strong as the abdominal muscles."[5]
"I condemn the wholesale prescription of flexion routines."[13]

Studies show that patients with back pain do not have abnormally weak abdominals, but instead have relatively weak extensor muscles.[10] Flexion is contraindicated for patients with acute disk problems; it contributes to the motion of the disk's nucleus toward prolapse. In the morning, because the disks have absorbed more fluid during sleep, flexion exercises can result in 300 percent more stress on the lumbar disks than the same movements later in the day.[2] Patients with posturally induced back pain from excessive sitting should also avoid flexion routines. Flexion may be the most helpful approach for some, but no patient should be handed a mimeographed sheet of Williams flexion exercises which presumably addresses all causes of back pain. Before attempting to strengthen or lengthen specific muscles, an evaluation should be done to determine which are weak or tight.

Muscles that Move the Spine

Abdominals

The stomach muscles flex the spine/trunk and provide the strength for such functions as coughing, straining and forced exhalation. The abdominals are composed of four individual muscles; the "rectus" runs vertically and performs straight flexion and the "obliques" run diagonally to perform flexion with rotation. [See Figure 9-1]

Spinal Muscles

The muscles of the spine consist of four muscle groups which attach to and connect the vertebrae. The "erector spinae" are referred to as the paravertebral, paraspinal or back extensor muscles; the fibers of this muscle group cross several vertebrae and perform the opposite motion to the abdominals - they extend the spine. [See Figure 9-1] They are responsible for maintaining an erect posture of the trunk against gravity.

Other smaller spinal muscles run between adjacent vertebrae. Their role is to steady the spinal column, preventing buckling between vertebrae. They provide stability at each vertebral joint, so that the erector spinae muscles can extend the whole spine in a smooth motion.

Muscles Crossing the Hip Joint

The hamstring muscles participate in hip and trunk extension and the gluteal muscles participate in hip and trunk hyperextension (extension past neutral). These two muscle groups provide the power for lifting from a flexed position. The hamstrings are the muscles which form the back of the thigh; their prime action is to flex the knee. The gluteals cover the back and sides of the pelvis, forming the bulk of the buttocks; their prime action is hip extension and abduction. [See Figure 9-1]

The hip flexor muscles assist the abdominals in trunk flexion in addition to flexing the hip joint. The bulk of the muscle is located inside the pelvis and can't easily be palpated.

Box 9-2

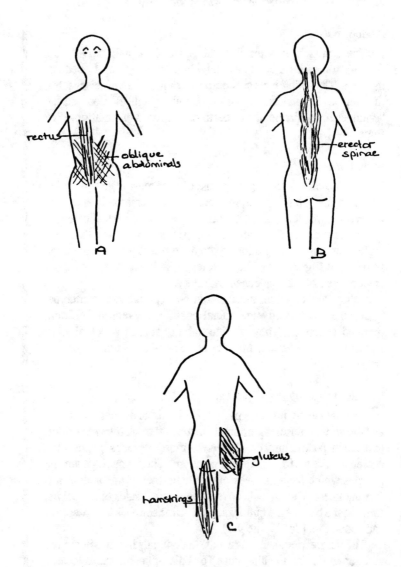

Figure 9-1. Muscles effecting the spine. (A) Abdominals (trunk flexion), front view. (B) Erector spinae (trunk extension), back view. (C) Hamstrings and gluteals (hip extension), back view.

Specific Flexion Exercises

Muscles which are strengthened by flexion exercises include the abdominals (rectus and obliques), gluteals and hip flexors. Muscles stretched by flexion exercises include spinal muscles (especially the erector spinae), hamstrings and hip flexors. [See Figure 9-1] [See Box 9-2]

1) **Valsalva's Maneuver** - Patients are often encouraged to learn to voluntarily contract the abdominals with a closed glottis, i.e. tightening the stomach muscles without exhaling, as in straining. This is meant to increase intra-abdominal pressure (IAP), protecting the spine during flexion. This voluntary contraction involves the rectus abdominal muscle; however, IAP is a reflex carried out by the obliques. It may not respond to conscious training. If voluntary abdominal contractions can improve reflex intra-abdominal pressure to protect the spine, then the obliques should be the abdominals to be targeted.[10]

2) **Abdominal Sets** - Tensing the abdominals with no resultant movement of the trunk is an isometric contraction. Because the joints of the spine don't move, this exercise produces relatively low stress on the back. It can be done and maintained with significant force to be effective as an abdominal strengthener.

3) **Gluteal Sets** - The gluteal muscles, which make up the bulk of the buttocks, are strengthened by squeezing the buttocks together and holding. This exercise is called a gluteal set. Tensing the gluteals flattens the lumbar curve or lordosis.

4) **Pelvic Tilts** - Pelvic tilts, which flatten the lumbar lordosis, strengthen the abdominals as well as the gluteal muscles. The pelvic tilt in backlying with knees bent is one of the best flexion exercises for involving the abdominal obliques while minimizing flexion of the low back.[6,10] With legs extended, the rectus muscle is excessively involved. In standing, increased activity of back extensor muscles occurs. Sciatica can be aggravated by contraction of the gluteal muscles during the pelvic tilt. The backlying pelvic tilt decreases EMG activity in the spinal muscles (erector spinae); in other words, this exercise can be effective in reducing spasm of the back muscles.[4]

5) **Straight Leg Raise** - In an SLR, (hip flexion with knee extension in backlying), most of the work is carried out by hip flexors, so it is not an efficient abdominal exercise. If the abdominals are not strong,

lordosis is increased and pressure on the disks increases by 150 percent.[3]

6) **Knees to Chest** - This exercise is used to stretch back extensors, decreasing the lumbar lordosis. However, the spinal muscles do not have the mechanical leverage to significantly increase lordosis and do not usually need to be lengthened.[10] When back extensors are in spasm, slowly bringing knees to chest may help relax the muscles.

7) **One Knee to Chest** - Tight hip flexors can increase lordosis; bringing one knee to the chest stretches the hip flexors of the opposite leg which remains extended.

8) **Toe Touch** - This is a hamstring stretching exercise; the hamstring muscles, when tight, are thought to overstretch and stress the lower spine during trunk flexion. A common hamstring stretch involves toe touching and bouncing. Toe touches cause a marked increase in pressure on the disks; bouncing causes reflex contraction of the muscle, negating the purpose of the exercise. The preferred method is to stretch only one leg at a time; this balances the lumbar spine. Keep one leg straight in either backlying or standing while flexing the opposite hip with the knee extended. Another method is to keep one knee to the chest while leaning forward in floor-sitting while the opposite leg remains flat on the floor.[5]

9) **Sit-ups** - Sit-ups of various kinds are one of the most common exercises performed, from children in gym class, to dieters, to patients with low back pain. It is also an exercise which generates a 210 percent increase in disk pressure.[3] Sit-ups can be done with arms forward or behind the head, raising just the head, coming completely to sitting, or anything in between. [See Figure 9-2]

- Sit-ups with legs fully extended exercise the hip flexors versus the abdominals, (for the first 30 degrees), displace the L-5 vertebra anteriorly over the sacrum and increase lordosis.[5]

- Sit-ups with hips and knees flexed increase the role of the abdominals somewhat and eliminate the lordosis, but still displace the L-5 vertebra.

- Many experts now recommend sit-ups never be done to the point of the low back leaving the floor; the trunk is raised only to the mid-back level (30 degrees) and held. Hip flexors still assist in this sit-up though the strain on the low back is considerably reduced.

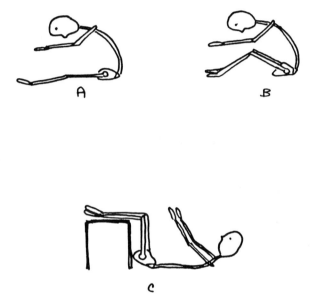

Figure 9-2. Sit-ups. (A) Full sit-up with extended knees. (B) Full sit-up with flexed knees. (C) Partial sit-up with flexed knees and lower legs supported and raised.

- A sit-up which eliminates use of hip flexors and avoids back pain is done with the hips and knees flexed up to 90 degrees with the calves resting on a chair seat; the body curls up to 45 degrees. The neck should be held in neutral to avoid neck discomfort.[1]
- A sit-back is a sit-up in reverse, or lengthening contraction of the abdominals; it is at least as effective in increasing strength.
- Diagonal sit-ups or sit-backs exercise the abdominal obliques, which should not be left out if promoting abdominal strength. Diagonal, partial sit-ups with knees flexed is one of the best flexion exercises for involving the obliques while minimizing lower spine flexion.[5]

Extension Exercises

Extension exercises can be divided into two categories, (1) those started from a flexed or neutral (straight) position to improve strength and endurance, and (2) those done in hyperextension (arching backwards past neutral) to improve mobility and promote a shift of nuclear material with a disk prolapse. The rationale for extension exercises is to . . .

- promote maintenance of normal spinal curves
- remove stress from the disks
- move the nucleus of a protruding disk centrally
- develop strength for lifting
- increase strength and endurance of spinal muscles, (which have been shown to be relatively weak in patients with back pain)
- minimize excessive flexion postures
- restore normal balance in which extensor should be stronger than flexor strength.

Extension exercises are contraindicated (1) in patients with acute disk rupture if they do not decrease symptoms, (2) for the multioperated back with disruption or scarring of posterior structures and (3) with certain structural abnormalities such as stenosis and spondylolisthesis.[10] Extension compresses the facet joints and narrows the openings between vertebrae; this may aggravate symptoms in patients with degenerative disease.

Specific Extension Exercises

Muscles which are strengthened by extension exercises include the spinal muscles (erector spinae and smaller stabilizing back muscles), gluteals and hamstrings. [See Figure 9-1] [See Box 9-2]

Active Extension/Postural Holding - The primary functions of the erector spinae are (1) postural holding and (2) control of trunk flexion through lengthening contractions. Maximum demand occurs at 40-45 degrees of trunk flexion, so the ideal exercise would begin working in this range with holding and a lengthening contraction incorporated. The smaller spinal muscles control the joints between adjacent vertebrae, preventing buckling between vertebrae during trunk extension. An exercise for these deep spinal muscles is on all fours with opposite arm and leg raised; the patient is gently pushed and pulled in different directions and has to stabilize the back to maintain balance.[12]

Passive Extension - Press-ups or backward bending in standing is used to reduce pain and protrusion from a bulging disk. This exercise does not actively exercise the extensors as the motion is carried out with the strength of the arms. [See Figure 9-3] It presupposes intact annular fibers and should not be done unless pain relief is obtained; even passive motion can stress the disk slightly.

Hip Extension - The hamstrings and gluteals participate in extension and hyperextension of both hip and trunk; these two muscle groups provide the power for lifting from a flexed position. Abnormally weak hams or gluts should be identified in examination and addressed in an exercise program. The hamstrings are exercised through resisted knee flexion and the gluteals through resisted hip extension.

The neck, as well as the low back, requires adequate strength and flexibility to minimize pain and risk of injury. The neck, like the trunk, moves in flexion, extension, lateral flexion and rotation. The chin tuck is a position which combines flexion at the joint between neck and skull with maintenance of the normal cervical lordosis; this position corrects the slumped, chin jutting posture which is so common. Musculature of the shoulder and upper back can influence neck posture and should be evaluated when designing an exercise program for neck pain.

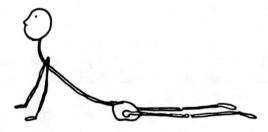

Figure 9-3. A "press-up"; passive hyperextension of the spine performed to relieve a prolapsed disk.

Exercise for Normal Movement Patterns

Isolated strengthening exercises may not address the problem of normal muscle function; muscle "skill" depends on the development of rapid, alternating contractions and relaxations, not just strength. During most activities, muscles must respond rapidly to maintain the body's center of gravity and for smooth efficient movement. Back pain may cause disuse, overuse or misuse of certain muscles, disrupting normal postural balance and movement patterns.[8,9]

One exercise program which emphasizes whole body movement patterns uses a large "Playball" to develop automatic responses to balance displacement.[8] Another incorporates the use of biofeedback so patients can relearn normal recruitment and relaxation of muscles for postural holding and active movement.[9] PNF, NDT, Feldenkrais, Rolfing and the Alexander Technique are therapeutic approaches which also address movement patterns; these are all discussed in PART 3, "Alternative Treatments for Back Pain."

During an acutely painful episode, regular exercises may need to be cut back; the patient can continue to be aware of proper posture/body mechanics, perform less stressful movements and then gradually resume the program. Progress can be monitored by the feedback received form the body; if an exercise increases pain, it should be modified or eliminated.[6] Many people with recurrent back problems report fewer and shorter episodes of pain if they stick to an individualized exercise program. Individualization of exercises is crucial; their selection should be based on an evaluation which addresses the effects of posture and movement on symptoms. The goal of an exercise program for people with back pain is to restore

- normal spinal curves,
- mobility of soft tissues and joints, and
- muscle strength, endurance and balance.[11]

Key Points - Back Exercises

Evidence supports the use of flexion or extension exercise programs in a select group of patients. However, their indications may be limited and the specific exercises used should be chosen carefully. Williams flexion exercises used to be prescribed for every patient with back pain, but it is now recognized that both flexion and extension strength are necessary for a healthy, posturally balanced spine. What is of utmost importance is that any effective exercise program has to be individualized. Descriptions, rationales, pros and cons for flexibility, strengthening, flexion and extension exercises are discussed in this chapter.

Footnotes

1   *The Back Letter*, Vol. 4, No. 3
2   *The Back Letter*, Vol. 4, No. 8
3   Glenna Batson, "Reeducating or Strengthening: Relooking at the Pelvic Tilt"
4   Blackburn & Portney, "Electromyographic Activity of Back Musculature During Williams' Flexion Exercises"
5   Rene Cailliet, *Low Back Pain Syndrome*
6   Deborah Caplan, *Back Trouble*
7   Charles Fager, "The Neurosurgical Management of Lumbar Spine Disease"
8   Barbara Headley, "Dynamic Stabilization"
9   Barbara Headley, "Postural Homeostasis"
10 Jackson & Brown, "Analysis of Current Approaches and a Practical Guide to Prescription of Exercise"
11 James McGavin, "The McKenzie Approach to Spinal Pain"
12 Stanley Paris, "Physical Signs of Instability"
13 Stanley Paris, *The Spine*

Chapter 10 - Physical Conditioning

"There is considerable evidence to support the fact that regular exercise is the single most important thing that you can do to have a healthy neck and back." Duane Saunders, PT[7]
"Aerobic conditioning seems to offer the most benefit to all kinds of back problems." Claudia Jackson, PT, & Mark Brown, MD[5]
"Most back pain patients are best advised to live with their disorder and fight it with activity." Charles Fager, MD[3]

It is well documented that the physically fit person is less likely to suffer a back injury and one of shorter duration if it does occur. Exercise can speed recovery and prevent injuries from recurring.[1] Excessive inactivity has been shown to have multiple harmful effects, as discussed in Chapter 4 under "Bedrest." Exercise, in whatever form, is considered to have multiple benefits.

- promotion of cardiovascular fitness
- maintenance of muscle strength and endurance
- increase of blood flow to injured tissues

- elongation of soft tissues (muscles, tendons, joint capsules and ligaments)
- pain inhibition
- promotion of mental well-being
- reduction of stress [See Box 10-1]

Exercise and Stress Reduction

Exercise is thought to stimulate the production of endorphins; these are morphine-like derivatives produced in the brain which are the body's natural pain-killers. Studies have found that exercises which do not increase the body's use of oxygen do not effect endorphin response. On the other hand, high intensity exercise results in a dramatic endorphin increase which falls off rapidly when exercise ceases. This indicates that high intensity exercise can raise pain tolerance, decrease pain sensation and elevate mood.[4] (This is one explanation of the "runner's high.") Another theory is that moderate exercise increases metabolism and uses up excess "catecholamines"; these are compounds produced by the body as a response to stress. Intense exercise, however, releases more catecholamines.[2]

Box 10-1

To optimize physical conditioning, "aerobic" exercises should be selected. Aerobic exercises are so called because they (1) increase the body's use of oxygen and (2) increase heart and lung activity through rhythmic, repetitive activities lasting over 20 minutes. Examples of aerobic exercises are running, walking, swimming, dancing and biking. As with other activities of daily living, posture and body mechanics should be considered before choosing a physical conditioning program.

Guidelines for Physical Conditioning
- Individuals with recurrent back problems should resume aerobic activities after a relatively pain-free interval of 2 weeks. (This advice is not for patients restricted due to a systemic disease or

those recovering from a traumatic injury.)

- Sessions should range from 20-40 minutes and include warmup and cool-down periods.
- 3 to 5 sessions weekly are necessary to achieve the full benefits of exercise while minimizing the risk of injury.
- Activities should increase heart and breathing rates and involve large muscle groups.
- Temperature extremes should be avoided.
- New exercise programs should start slowly with a gradual increase in the number and difficulty of activities.
- The activity should not cause pain that lingers after the activity stops.

Physical Conditioning Activities

Walking, most experts agree, is a beneficial and recommended activity for those with back pain. Good shoes are advised.

Swimming is a non-weight bearing activity, so causes the least amount of stress on disks and joints. Stroke selection can be made to emphasize flexion or extension. However, an unskilled swimmer may assume poor postures with inefficient use of energy. Cold water temperature, the expense and driving distance to a pool may create problems for some back pain patients.

Jogging, some say, does not necessarily stress spinal structures, but others are concerned about the effects on disks and weight-bearing joints. Unskilled joggers may assume poor postures with inefficient use of energy. Good shoes are necessary for this activity.

Biking may not be ideal for some people due to the prolonged flexion position of the spine when sitting on a bicycle. Seat and handle bar height should be adjusted for optimum comfort.

Exercise classes include gym workouts, dance, aerobics classes, jazzercise and a large variety of fitness oriented programs. The YMCA, for example, has a back program of relaxation, flexibility and strengthening exercises which they claim improves 80 percent of participants and cures 31 percent.[9] Activities such as jump rope can cause repetitive over-loading on spinal structures; exercise classes may require excessive twisting and forward bending. People with back problems should use caution in signing up for fitness classes. Instructors for these programs have varying qualifications and experience. Both the program and the instructor should be evaluated to be sure that individualization can be incorporated into the program without pressure on the participant to keep up with the class.

In Klein and Sobel's survey of chronic pain patients, the most successful approaches to providing "dramatic long-term help" were found to be physical conditioning activities. Dance therapy, fitness classes and yoga were among the few treatment approaches with 50 percent or more of respondents achieving this level of success.[6] However, the benefits applied to individuals not severely incapacitated by back pain. Yoga, fitness classes and dance may be too strenuous for people with certain back conditions.

Chronic back pain and its adjustments can cause a measurable reduction in physical fitness; this can be reversed in a short time with a simple, individualized activity program.[8]

Key Points - Physical Conditioning

Physical conditioning is beneficial for everyone - to prevent back problems or relapses, minimize the number and duration of acute episodes, speed recovery and reduce pain. To avoid causing injury and to provide the most benefits, an exercise program should be specifically designed to meet individual needs. It is important for people with back pain to find the activity level appropriate to their disabilities.

Footnotes

1 *The Back Letter,* "Memo on Body Mechanics"
2 Pat Croce, "Put Stress to Rest"
3 Charles Fager, "The Neurosurgical Management of Lumbar Spine Disease"
4 Billy Glisan, et al., "Physiology of Active Exercise in Rehabilitation of Back Injuries"
5 Jackson & Brown, "Is There a Role for Exercise in the Treatment of Patients with Low Back Pain"
6 Klein & Sobel, *Backache Relief*
7 Duane Saunders, *For Your Neck*
8 Lynn Thomas, et al., "Physiological Work Performance in Chronic Low Back Disability"
9 Judith Willis, "Back Pain: Ubiquitous, Controversial"

Chapter 11 - Special Programs

Work Hardening

"Employment is nature's physician, and is essential to human happiness." Galen

Individuals whose back injuries have left them unable to perform their job duties should return to work as soon as possible.[6] Staying out of work promotes general weakness and adverse psychological effects. The benefits of physical activity and harmful effects of inactivity are numerous, as discussed in Chapter 4 under "Bedrest" and in Chapter 10, "Physical Conditioning."

Work hardening programs, also called "functional restoration," are for the injured worker; they are frequently offered by Physical and Occupational Therapy departments. Their goal is to provide rehabilitation specifically geared toward an individual's work place; this promotes the worker's prompt and safe return to the job. Various factors affect a worker's ability to successfully return to work. These include ...

- characteristics of the job, such as the demand for lifting, the need for awkward or sustained postures and whole body vibration
- previous physical conditioning of the employee
- mental attitude of the employee toward the job
- mental attitude of the employer toward the worker and the worker's injury.

The job site or equipment/tools may have to be adapted to meet an injured worker's needs; this is what is meant by the term "ergonomics". The worker also has to adapt by learning new, safer work habits and making them a permanent part of the job.

Guidelines for Work Hardening Programs

- Intervene early to begin rehabilitation and accustom the worker to the idea of returning to work.
- Determine if the worker has concerns, misleading or confusing information, or unrealistic expectations concerning workers' compensation laws. Fear can be misinterpreted as malingering and needs to be addressed.
- Make it clear that the worker is responsible for participating in his/her own rehabilitation.
- Draw up a written agreement stating the purpose, goals and expectations of therapy and the criteria for discharge.
- Set time goals with the worker.
- Compare a worker's capabilities to the physical demands of the workplace.
- Simulate the work-place by stressing work related activities; recondition the worker using the tools and postures used on the job. This encourages confidence and the mindset that he/she can and will return to work.
- Develop a schedule which sets an appropriate work pace, not so fast that symptoms are increased and not so slow that return to work is unnecessarily delayed.
- Alternate activity with relaxation and keep increasing activity level until the worker can participate in a regular work setting.

- Educate the worker about his/her injury and how to prevent a recurrence.
- Observe the worker performing actual work tasks before he/she returns to a less supervised setting.

An early return to the job can often prevent chronic pain from developing; when a worker focuses on productive work rather than pain, there is less tendency for pain related personality traits to develop. When the health practitioner and employer act as advocates rather than adversaries for the injured worker, the worker's confidence and motivation to return to work can be improved. Work hardening is a way to increase a worker's chances for returning to the job and to reduce the risk of reinjury.

Pain Clinics

"There are disastrous side effects from pain because we focus on relief from a pain which usually has no clear cause and no clear cure; the real problem is not the pain, but how we handle it." Edward Abraham, MD[1]

Pain clinics are multidisciplinary centers offering a combination of physical therapy, occupational therapy, psychological testing, counseling, social work, pharmacology, vocational counseling, nursing and a variety of specializing physicians. Such clinics are effective because all the necessary treatment approaches are in one place at one time; fewer medical work-ups are needed and more options available. The major factor required is the patient's willing cooperation. Most people with chronic pain are said to have difficulties with drugs, dependence, depression, anxiety and/or physical deconditioning. The role of the clinic is to detoxify from drug use, to desensitize to pain perception, to provide relaxation training, basic exercises and physical conditioning and to teach patients to take an active role in managing their pain.[4,12] The goal is not to cure, but to give patients the ability to live with their disabilities.[9]

The philosophy of pain clinics varies; what governs the specific approach is most likely the director's specialty.[12] [See Box 11-1]

Specific Pain Clinics

1) At the University of Miami center, chronic pain patients work through their pain; they are pushed to the limit, building up to rigorous physical training and exercise. The emphasis is on coping and functioning with the pain versus eliminating it.[12]

2) At Folsom Physical Therapy, the underlying premise is that pain causes no gain; the first step is to find the positions that cause pain and avoid them. The patient is then taught to be pain-free in all activities and learns to have control by being able to avoid painful positions.[10]

3) In the Casa Colina Program of Pain Management, the emotional/mental components of pain are recognized as crucial elements in the whole picture; the patient is expected to give up the invalid role and is taught assertiveness skills.[7]

4) A clinic in Stony Brook, New York, relies on a new machine which shows the precise degree of muscle exertion produced during exercise. It is used to monitor progress and to motivate patients to build muscle strength. It also supposedly provides evidence of whether a person is exaggerating pain; a correlation is assumed between muscle exertion and pain production.[12]

Box 11-1

A comprehensive pain program usually includes the following services:
- drug control or prescription
- rehabilitation specifically aimed at the disability
- posture and body mechanics
- exercises for strength and flexibility
- pacing instruction to teach appropriate rest/activity balance
- physical reconditioning
- relaxation techniques (biofeedback, hypnosis, visualization)
- modification of how pain is perceived
- pain inhibition (TENS, acupuncture)
- psychological counseling
- stress management
- assertiveness training
- vocational evaluation, counseling and rehabilitation
- nutrition

Pain Coping Skills

Learning to cope with chronic pain is emphasized at many pain clinics. Emotional factors, environmental reinforcement and secondary gains can perpetuate a patient's pain. People can become victims to the pain, feeling trapped, threatened and unable to change.[8] The goal of pain management techniques is to replace pain-perpetuating behaviors with new coping behaviors. Instead of waiting to take up life where it left off, patients are encouraged to make adjustments to their disabilities and to resume an active life.[11] Pain clinics attempt to put the patient in charge. When a back problem becomes chronic, more and more responsibility for health care falls upon the patient. It is the patient who ultimately has the responsibility for managing the pain, finding alternative employment, selecting the most appropriate treatment approaches and learning how to resume and maintain an active lifestyle.[2,4,11]

Practitioners have various strategies to help their chronic pain patients develop the inner resources necessary for successful pain management.

1) Reassure the patient that the pain is not malignant or life-threatening; address his concerns. The chances for successful coping are improved if the patient is not overly anxious.

2) Be frank and tell the patient that the condition is not likely to change; the pain will have to be endured.[11] Change the patient's focus from finding a cure to managing the pain.

3) Teach the patient to alter the way pain is perceived. When pain is controlling one's life, it is seen as a warning, a danger signal and a barrier to activity. Pain eventually becomes synonymous with movement. A patient can learn to discriminate between activity and pain; if he accepts the pain as given, he can experience it while being active instead of having the same experience while being an invalid.[1,4,8]

4) Help the patient develop self-reliance and coping skills; there are many treatment approaches that promote relaxation, confidence or a positive outlook.

5) Offer the patient specific guidelines for successful coping.[4]

- Keep active and occupied.
- Direct yourself outward.
- Maintain a schedule compatible with the rest of the family and the world.
- Avoid advertising your suffering.

- Carry out an exercise routine suited to your needs.
- Commit yourself to a healthy lifestyle despite the hurt.
- Aim for the acceptance of pain without emotional distress.

As is true of any therapeutic approach, pain clinics must individualize their programs to be successful. Pain clinics are highly rated by some experts because they provide diagnosis from a broad perspective and offer many different treatments. One author advises anyone with pain that lasts more than 2 months to contact a comprehensive pain clinic, but reports that only 3 percent of Americans with chronic pain do so.[5] However, another author reports that intensive programs for people with chronic pain may have only short-term success; one study showed that after six months, the results were only partly maintained.[3]

Key Points - Special Programs

Work hardening programs provide rehabilitation for injured workers that is specifically geared toward activities performed on the job. The goal is to return individuals to work more promptly and safely, preventing the development of chronic pain and disability and minimizing the chances for reinjury.

Pain clinics are multidisciplinary centers which offer a wide range of diagnostic and treatment options for chronic pain. People with chronic back pain are helped to learn pain coping and management techniques and encouraged to resume an active lifestyle.

Footnotes

1 Edward Abraham, *Freedom From Back Pain: An Orthopedist's Guide*
2 "Approaches to Musculoskeletal Problems" Symposium, Jane Derebery
3 *The Back Letter*, Vol. 4, No. 3
4 Steven Brena, *Chronic Pain: America's Hidden Epidemic*
5 Jean Carper, *Health Care, U.S.A.*
6 Derebery & Tullis, "Delayed Recovery in the Patient with a Work Compensable Injury"
7 Harold Gottlieb, et al., "An Innovative Program for the Restoration of Patients with Chronic Back Pain"
8 Barbara Headley, "Pain Vs. Suffering"
9 Patricia McPhee, "Chronic Pain and the Role of Occupational Therapy"
10 Edith Montgomery, "Folsom Physical Therapy - A Different Approach to Back Rehabilitation"
11 Richard Sternbach, *Pain Patients: Traits and Treatments*
12 David Zinman, "Focus on Back Pain"

Chapter 12 - Manual Therapy

"Manipulation can provide dramatic relief of pain, spasm and restriction of motion." Paul Kaplan, MD, & Ellen Tanner, PT[12]

"Many patients do report dramatic relief, others recover despite manipulation." Charles Fager, MD[10]

Manual therapy is the use of the hands to bring about therapeutic changes within the body. Manipulation and mobilization are the two major categories of manual therapy. Other forms of manual therapy include massage, (covered in Chapter 7), and myofascial treatments, (covered in Chapters 13 and 14). Manipulation under anesthesia is discussed in Chapter 6, "Surgery."

Manipulation

Manipulation is a sudden thrust applied to a joint to correct a dysfunction at that joint; it is of high velocity and small amplitude. Also called a spinal adjustment, manipulation is performed too quickly for the patient to control. The practitioner first moves a joint to the limits of its available mobility; then a sudden thrust ruptures adhesions and takes the joint beyond its normal range, but without exceeding its structural limits.[15,19] A specific thrust frees one joint in one direction in one maneuver.

Manipulation is used by both osteopaths and chiropractors to treat patients with back pain. However, not only do their manipulative techniques differ, but their philosophies as well. Osteopaths manipulate to correct a dysfunctional state of muscles and chiropractors to restore normal bony alignment. Because their views on the cause of back pain differ, so do their treatment methods. [See Box 12-1]

Manipulative Techniques

Osteopaths manipulate by localizing their force at the level of impaired mobility; thrust is applied with the minimum force necessary, usually in the direction of limitation. If the limitation is too great, more gentle techniques are used. The patient is positioned so that the joints on either side of the hypomobile segment are locked through ligament tension or facet joint position. A thrust is then imparted to restore mobility to that segment.[7,19]

Chiropractors palpate for vertebral displacement rather than decreased mobility. They apply pressure to the bone itself, using force to shift the vertebra back into place.[7] Unlike the protective locking used by osteopaths, pressure is applied to vertebral bony processes in order to open the space between the vertebrae; a high velocity thrust is then delivered to realign the segment.[19]

Box 12-1

A popping or cracking sound often accompanies manipulation. This may be caused by the breaking of an adhesion. Another cause is a pressure change when joint surfaces are suddenly forced apart. A carbon dioxide gas bubble, liberated from the synovial fluid inside the joint space, collapses with a crack.[15,19]

Mobilization

Mobilization is performed within a patient's available range of motion and is of lower speed and amplitude than manipulation. Mobilization techniques involve graded, gentle, rhythmic movements at specific joints, done within the patient's tolerance. The joint is passively taken to the limit of its available range where a series of gentle stretches or progressive reciprocal movements are performed to gradually relieve restriction.[19] Mobilization is also used for freeing soft tissue restrictions.

Manual Therapy: Therapeutic Effects

There are different schools of thought as to the specific effects that manual therapy has on the body. Treatment may be applied to address any one of the following:

1) joint or movement dysfunction
2) nerve root compression
3) pain
4) soft tissue restrictions
5) disease of a body system or organ.

Manual Therapy for Joint/Movement Dysfunction

Mennell first emphasized the importance of the small involuntary movements within a joint called "joint play"; he saw its loss as the basis for movement dysfunctions.[14,20] Stanley Paris believes that loss of joint play, in the facet joints specifically, is the primary cause of back pain and dysfunction. He treats patients with mobilization techniques to restore joint mobility.[19] Joint mobilization is indicated when there is a loss of joint play due to tightness or adhesions of soft tissues which surround a joint, (i.e. joint capsule, connective tissue and ligaments). In cases where tissue is pinched between the joint surfaces, a maneuver in flexion is used to separate the joint and free the trapped structure.

Manipulation or mobilization of the sacroiliac joint is the preferred treatment for SIJ dysfunction. Significant improvement is obtained when a specific maneuver is used to correct an entrapped sacrum.[2]

Manual Therapy for Nerve Root Compression

James Cyriax pioneered the use of manipulation for disk problems; he considered disks to be the primary site of spinal pain.[3] Rather than restoring mobility, Cyriax's techniques are based on moving a small fragment of disk. Maneuvers are carried out during strong traction, separating the joint and giving the fragment room to move.[7] Traction also creates suction to pull the disk fragment and tightens the posterior longitudinal ligament to push the fragment back into place. Enough force is applied to take up the slack in the affected area, then a sudden manipulative thrust moves the displaced fragment and frees any adhesions around the disk.

The biggest concern in the use of manipulation to relieve nerve root compression is the possibility of serious neurological consequences. Some patients with disk pathology have developed neurologic signs following manipulation, indicating that the treatment worsened the condition.[10] Many experts recommend that patients with nerve root compression be excluded from this kind of treatment; they also favor eliminating those with involvement of spinal cord, cauda equina, nerve roots, vertebral arteries and disease of vertebrae or spinal ligaments.[17] Gentle nonrotary mobilizations are thought safe, but it is uncertain whether disk protrusions are helped by manual therapy.[12] After the acute phase of a disk prolapse, mobilization may be beneficial to maintain mobility at the affected segment.[13]

Manual Therapy for Pain Relief
Two manual therapy pioneers, Maigne and Maitland, used mobilization for pain relief. Maigne felt that if a procedure is painful, it shouldn't be done; if a joint is stiff in one direction, he recommended freeing it by moving it in the direction of its greatest mobility.[19] Maitland also worked within pain tolerance, using a series of front-to-back repetitive, rhythmic thrusts; amplitude and force were varied to meet the demands of the condition.[19]

Manual therapy is thought to relieve pain in at least two ways.

1) It may stimulate the production of endorphins, (the body's own pain-killers); high levels are reported after treatment.

2) The sensory stimulation produced by manipulative techniques inhibits pain perception. Sensory messages from nerve endings in ligaments and joint capsules travel faster than slower pain messages. Stimulating these nerve fibers through manual therapy therefore blocks pain transmission.

Manual Therapy for Soft Tissue Effects
MDs tend to consider manipulation a treatment that primarily breaks down joint adhesions and relieves muscle spasm.[11]

1) Muscle spasm can be relieved through "reflex inhibition". A manipulative thrust desensitizes the nerve endings in a joint capsule; the muscle no longer receives a message to contract tightly to protect the joint. This is vastly preferable to forcibly moving a joint through protective muscle

spasm.

2) Another soft tissue effect of manual therapy is an increase in the patient's flexibility; manipulation can stretch or break contracted structures. Adhesions are put on maximum strain while other joint structures are on slack; adhesions are brittle and will break more easily with a sudden thrust than if allowed to elongate slowly.[19]

3) Ligament sprain may also be affected by manipulation; improperly formed scar tissue is torn, giving the ligament a chance to heal more strongly in proper alignment.[4]

Manual Therapy for Systemic Diseases

Mobilization is used by chiropractors and osteopaths for its effects on the organs of the body and for the general treatment of disease. This is discussed in Chapter 2 under "Osteopathic Doctors" and "Chiropractors."

Manual Therapy: Evaluation Methods

Just as practitioners have different reasons for performing manual therapy, they also use different diagnostic methods for recommending treatment and evaluating progress. There are pitfalls associated with each approach and the skilled practitioner needs to be knowledgeable about the pros and cons of each. Manual therapy may be recommended based on ...

1) pain
2) functional mobility
3) structural asymmetry, or
4) x-rays

Pain

Some studies which assess manipulation/mobilization claim 80 percent success, based on reports of pain after treatment.[9] These are difficult studies to compare as they vary in combining manipulation with other forms of treatment, in types of patients excluded, in techniques and in assessment tools used. Because of all the factors discussed in Chapter 1 under "Normal Pain," pain is a very unreliable symptom by which to monitor treatment.

Functional Mobility

Functional improvement is considered by many to be a much more reliable guide to progress than pain.[19] However, when function is the only measure of progress, manipulation may be continued past the time of pain relief. This can result in excessive treatment causing hypermobility, decreasing stability and leading to degenerative changes.[17] (One can get a similar effect from excessively "cracking" one's own back, which can eventually increase instability.)[19]

Structural Asymmetry

Manipulators often base treatment on asymmetry within the spinal column or variations in mobility between spinal segments; this is determined by "palpation," or examination through touch. Asymmetry, however, is very common and often found in people without pain.[18] What is considered an abnormality on palpation may be a normally functioning joint, i.e. one with its joint surfaces perfectly opposed.[18] There is a poor association between sites thought to be the origin of pain by palpation and areas of poor functional mobility.[18]

X-rays

Treatment based solely on x-ray results can be inappropriate. Many people with asymmetries, abnormalities or degenerative changes are pain free. When seen on x-ray, these postural asymmetries or painfree spinal abnormalities are often diagnosed as subluxations. These "subluxations" may then be unnecessarily treated. X-rays are recommended by many, not to identify sites appropriate for treatment, but to determine if there are contraindications to treatment.[12,17]

Manipulation: Limitations and Precautions

Manipulation can produce dramatic, positive results for some back pain patients. Practitioners who use manipulation explain its success as a result of . . .

- correction of a vertebral subluxation
- correction of a somatic dysfunction
- restoration of joint play
- displacement of a disk fragment
- stretching of a tight muscle
- tearing of soft tissue adhesions, or

- relief of muscle spasm.

There is no definitive proof that any of these is correct.[6]

Manipulation's scientific rationale is unconvincing to many.[8] Some believe that when manipulation appears to reduce pain it is due to the laying on of hands, temporary pain inhibition, the self-limiting nature of most illnesses, or the placebo effect. There is psychological value in the laying on of hands and the offer of a sympathetic ear in a non-hurried atmosphere, (unlike that found in many medical offices). Patients who have been unable to receive a firm diagnosis elsewhere are reassured to put themselves into the hands of someone who is confident about the cause of pain and the appropriate treatment. The placebo effect depends on inspiring this confidence.

A number of practitioners feel that high velocity thrust is inappropriate for most spinal conditions and that most patients do better with mobilization. These experts recommend that manipulation not be used at the beginning of treatment and never with a very painful joint or a joint being protected by muscle spasm. It may be appropriate for certain patients to later progress from mobilizations to manipulations.[17] Manipulation is a treatment that can involve risks. It should not be used with conditions such as osteoporosis, bone tumors, infection of spinal structures or hemorrhage.[7,12] Stroke symptoms or vertebral artery blockage (even leading to death) have been associated with manipulation.[12] Many of the patients whose spinal pain can't be diagnosed may be well suited for manipulation, but treatment should be related to symptoms and based on an evaluation of both function and structure. It is unwise to manipulate a joint merely because it hurts and there are no apparent contraindications.

There should be an immediate change in mobility or pain level with manipulation; if relief is not obtained within about three treatments, manipulations will probably not be effective.[1,4,11] A general rule for practitioners who use manipulation/mobilization is to use the gentlest technique which will produce the desired results.[17] An increasingly widely held view is that manipulation has positive short-term effects for some, especially when combined with other treatments, but that long-term benefits are questionable.[5,9,16] In other words, manipulation may speed improvement but doesn't affect the long-term prognosis for many back patients.

There is no doubt that manipulation/mobilization is not a cure-all. It is unfortunate that practitioners have made exaggerated claims about its benefits, but also that orthodox medicine tends to dismiss manual therapy in cases where it would be helpful.

Key Points - Manual Therapy

Manipulation and mobilization are used to relieve nerve root compression, relieve pain, normalize joint mobility and/or release soft tissue restrictions. Practitioners may recommend manual therapy based on pain, structural asymmetry, functional mobility or x-rays; probably all these factors should be taken into account. Many in the field of back pain express concern regarding the safety and effectiveness of manipulation. They feel that mobilization techniques are preferable to more vigorous manipulation and are as effective. They recommend using the gentlest form of manual therapy which produces positive results. Manipulation alone seems to help some patients, but often does not produce long-term relief. If manipulation is going to be successful for an individual patient, pain and mobility should noticeably improve within about three treatments.

Footnotes

1   "Approaches to Musculoskeletal Problems: Focus on the Low Back" Symposium, Donald Fraser
2   *The Back Letter*, Vol. 4, No. 2
3   *The Back Letter*, Vol. 4, No. 4
4   Ben Benjamin, "The Mystery of Lower Back Pain"
5   Rene Cailliet, *Low Back Pain Syndrome*
6   Consumer Reports Books, *Health Quackery*
7   James Cyriax, *Textbook of Orthopaedic Medicine*
8   Richard Deyo, "Conservative Therapy for Low Back Pain"
9   Richard DiFabio, "Clinical Assessment of Manipulation and Mobilization of the Lumbar Spine"
10 Charles Fager, "Beware the Quick Fix for Back Pain"
11 David Imrie, *Goodbye Back Ache*
12 Kaplan & Tanner, *Musculoskeletal Pain and Disability*
13 Randolph Kessler, "Acute Symptomatic Disk Prolapse"
14 Kessler & Hertling, *Management of Common Musculoskeletal Disorders*
15 W.H. Kirkaldy-Willis, *Managing Low Back Pain*
16 Klein & Sobel, *Backache Relief*
17 G.D. Maitland, *Vertebral Manipulation*
18 James McGavin, "The McKenzie Approach to Spinal Pain"
19 Stanley Paris, *The Spine*
20 Duane Saunders, *Evaluation, Treatment and Prevention of Musculoskeletal Disorders*

PART 3 - ALTERNATIVE TREATMENTS FOR BACK PAIN

Chapter 13 - Fascia Based Treatments

"Myofascial release is performed by a very large number of respected physical therapists and physicians across our nation producing excellent clinically reproducible results daily." John Barnes, PT[2]

"I feel that such a proposed explanation for the basis of these [myofascial] techniques is at best laughable and at worst detrimental to the professional standing of physical therapy in the medical community." Richard Bunch, PT[6]

The soft tissues of the spine are usually defined to include muscles, tendons, ligaments, joint capsules and fascia (connective tissue). The importance of the fascia in health problems has recently gained popularity. Fascia, the largest and most pervasive organ system of the human body, exists below

119

the skin, around and infused with all structures and organs; it joins the whole body, even at the cellular level. Each muscle and organ develops in its sack of fascia which then connects to other muscle groups and organs. The brain and spinal cord are also covered by fascial type membranes, the three meninges; the tough outer membrane, the dura, attaches to the inside of the skull and spinal column. Fascia is thought to have many functions:

- ensheathing and supporting the muscles
- transmitting and determining movement
- participating in fluid exchange for physiological balance
- conducting electrical currents that give information to the surrounding cells.[11,12]

In response to an orthopedic injury, the fascia shortens and thickens; this causes dehydration and a corresponding loss in electrical conductivity. Fascia is likewise affected by stress; if stress-related postures and movement patterns persist, extra fascia will be built up and will hold these dysfunctional positions.[12]

The possible non-mechanical, psychological and bioelectrical properties of fascia play a big role in several controversial approaches to the treatment of back pain; the ones discussed here include cranial osteopathy, craniosacral therapy, myofascial release and somatoemotional release. (Rolfing also stresses the importance of fascia in health problems; it is covered in the next chapter, "Movement Reeducation.")

Cranial Osteopathy

Cranial Osteopathy was formulated within the osteopathic profession in the 1930s; its main principle is that life is maintained by three different body rhythms - lung respiration, heart circulation and the flow of cerebrospinal fluid.[10] Cerebrospinal fluid fills the space between the two inner meninges, providing protection and shock absorption for the brain and spinal cord. During inhalation, there is movement of the cranial (skull) bones. Because the skull lining (the dura) also lines the spinal column, movement of the skull bones causes movement of the spinal column and sacrum. In other words, breathing is reflected in the bones of the head and spine; the rhythm can be detected as minute pulsations called the craniosacral rhythm. Deviations from normal can be corrected through manipulation. A minority of osteopaths currently accept this concept.[10]

A small but growing number of chiropractors also regard musculoskeletal problems as secondary to the subtle rhythmic pulsing of the cerebrospinal fluid contained within the meninges.

"In health, all functions of the body are synchronized with the craniosacral rhythm."[9]

Various factors can impede the smooth flow of energy through the meninges and cerebro-spinal fluid. (One such factor is thought to be a diet too high in fats.[9]) When energy flow is disrupted, it interferes with the craniosacral rhythm and eventually causes mechanical distortion in the meninges. This, in turn, results in compression of the spinal cord, abnormal movement patterns and distorted alignment of the vertebrae. The end result, vertebral joints which lock up and lose function, are what chiropractors call subluxations. These mechanical distortions can also elicit various psychological patterns; the more abnormal the spine, the more emotional stress is created.[9]

Correction of subluxations through manipulation is the heart of the chiropractic profession. The meningeal theory is a point of contention for chiropractors because it does not consider subluxations as the ultimate cause of health problems.[9] Most chiropractors perform manipulation on the vertebral column at the site of subluxations; meningeal therapists emphasize cranial adjustments.

Craniosacral Therapy
Promoted by John Upledger, **craniosacral therapy** emphasizes normalization of the bones and meninges surrounding the brain and spinal cord to restore health. The craniosacral system is thought to generate a rhythm or pulse of 6-12 times/minute due to cyclical production of cerebro-spinal fluid. This rhythm can be detected, especially at the sacrum and base of the skull. Binding of the fascia around the spinal column affects bony movement; since the lining of the spinal column is continuous with the lining of the cranial bones, restricted movement of the spinal column affects cerebro-spinal fluid production. The result is pain, dysfunction and loss of a sense of well-being.[1,2] By palpating the sacrum and cranial bones, a therapist can evaluate the amplitude, rate, quality and strength of craniosacral movement. After detecting restrictions, gentle pressure is applied to release soft tissue, with beneficial effects on the patient's muscle tone, posture, bony alignment and emo-

tional state.[7] Craniosacral therapy, often performed by PTs, is a controversial treatment within the physical therapy profession.

Myofascial Release

John Barnes' **myofascial release**, often performed by physical therapists, treats dysfunction in the fascial system to increase soft tissue flexibility. Barnes claims that 90 percent of patients seen in physical therapy, and an extremely high percentage of those with pain, have myofascial dysfunction.[1,3] Myofascial dysfunction is a binding down of fascia due to trauma, faulty posture or inflammation; it causes pressure on nerves, muscles, bones and organs. Any fascial problem can lead to poor cellular efficiency, disease, pain or dysfunction throughout the body. Barnes says that this treatment approach has clinically reproducible results superior to those of conventional treatment.[2]

"Millions upon millions of desperate people are suffering now who need myofascial release."[2]

Somato-Emotional Release

The fascia's link with an individual's emotions is the focus in **somato-emotional release** or **myofascial unwinding**, an extension of myofascial release theory. Health problems permeate both mind and body and fascia is seen as a possible link between the two. Relieving fascial restrictions produces physiological reactions of the whole body, such as shaking, tremors or emotional outbursts. Fascial manipulation can tap into a person's subjective experiences and feelings. In the therapy setting, a safe environment to let go in, the patient who is freed from physical restrictions also experiences past traumatic experiences which are said to be stored in the fascia. This release allows the patient to gain insights into the mind/body restrictions which may be stopping full recovery.[6,7]

"Bioenergetics" is an approach that supports somato-emotional release theory. Its creator, Alexander Lowen, submits that the body is the repository of all experience; the influences that shape a person's character also shape physical structure, posture and style of moving and breathing. When a therapist works with the body, the recall of repressed memories and feelings is facilitated; touching the body has the potential for tapping into blocked, unresolved emotions.[8]

Critics of myofascial release, craniosacral therapy and similar approaches say that they are based on "completely unscientific quasi-transcendental dogma".[6] These techniques incorporate relaxation techniques and therapeutic manual pressure, as do many other therapies. Manual therapy and relaxation can produce pain relief associated with the production of endorphins and the placebo effect; this alone may explain the effectiveness of any therapy which incorporates them. The reported links to vague concepts such as energy flow and metaphysical theory are thought by many to cause physical therapy to lose respect as a profession based on clear scientific principles.[5]

"De-emphasizing 'methodical, scientific reasoning' as a foundation to our clinical approaches puts our profession in the same category as non-licensed, non-regulated charlatans." [4]

Myofascial restrictions can develop as the body's attempt to stabilize and protect an injured area. Treatment which removes myofascial restrictions may increase instability and pain if the cause of the original problem is not also addressed. Practitioners should formulate a plan to build functional stability before starting treatment to reduce the dysfunctional stability.

Key Points - Fascia Based Treatments

Fascia is the connective tissue of the body. It can thicken and restrict movement in response to injury or stress, and then perpetuate pain by holding the dysfunctional positions. The four approaches discussed in this chapter are based on the role of fascia and the craniosacral rhythm on pain and dysfunction. Manipulation of fascial restrictions and of the bones of the skull and sacrum is performed. This is thought to restore normal alignment, energy flow, soft tissue mobility and even to free unresolved emotions. The theory behind these approaches has caused significant controversy among health professionals. Before performing myofascial release, practitioners should consider whether their treatments could increase instability or trauma to the area.

Footnotes

1 John Barnes, "Benefits of Myofascial Release, Craniosacral Therapy Explained"
2 John Barnes, "Pro: Never Trademarked Myofascial Release"
3 John Barnes, "Therapeutic Insight"
4 Benanti & Ellis, "Holistic Medicine a 'Crisis' for PTs"
5 Ben Benjamin, "The Mystery of Lower Back Pain"
6 Richard Bunch, "Con: Myofascial Release Traced Back Decades"
7 Steve Heinrich, "Body Watch: The importance of Dialogue and Myofascial Unwinding in Creating a Safe Place to Heal"
8 Joyce Lauterback, "The Mind-Body Connection - Is There More?"
9 Mark Mead, "Chiropractic's New Wave"
10 Mills & Finando, *Alternatives in Healing*
11 Ida Rolf, "Structural Integration"
12 Michael Shea, "MFR and the Psychosomatic Body"
13 Weiselfish & Kain, "Introduction of Developmental Manual Therapy"

Chapter 14 - Movement Reeducation

Rolfing

"Adequate structure in the human is the basis for sound health, improved life and personal evolution." Rolf Institute Training Catalog

Rolfing was created by Ida Rolf and originally called Structural Integration; it treats victims of "the gravity disaster". Gravity is seen as the basic shaper of the body; when the body is properly aligned, the force of gravity can flow through it and promote self-healing. Rolfing seeks to organize the body so that the gravitational field can reinforce the body's energy field. This influences the individual's movement patterns, metabolism and psychology. When the major body parts are brought toward vertical alignment, this is experienced as a sense of lightness and increased energy level. The closer one gets to the vertical axis, the less gravity becomes a destructive force; energy is conserved for other purposes and long-term musculoskeletal deterioration is decreased.

Stress and pain are the body's expression of imbalance between gravity and body parts. Strain between body segments alters patterns of movement, restricting freedom of motion and draining energy. To achieve a balanced structure, the whole body must be treated, compensatory patterns as well as the areas that are targeted by a specific diagnosis.

The importance of fascia in health problems is emphasized in Rolfing. (Fascia's role and response to injury and stress are discussed in Chapter 13, "Fascia Based Treatments".) Fascia can support whatever postures the body adopts; with a physical injury it may thicken in an attempt to provide support, creating a chronic restriction. In Rolfing, fascial tissues are released and brought to a normal position; this is accomplished through manipulation, body education and appropriate movement patterns. Proper alignment depends on this balanced readjustment of fascial restrictions; it relieves stress and allows the body freedom to reorganize itself. These changes in structure are made permanent by the patient's ability to learn new movement patterns.[2,6,8]

Rolfers take a basic training course divided into two phases, Auditing and Practitioning, each comprising 324 hours. Prerequisites can be met in a 17-week course designed for entry into the program; they include kinesiology, massage, anatomy and psychology.

The Feldenkrais Method

"The time has come for humans to solve many of their personal health problems through a better use of their own brains." Frank Wildman, PhD[13]

The Feldenkrais Method is a treatment approach aimed at increasing a patient's sensory-motor awareness; the eventual goal is for more efficient and comfortable movement. Feldenkrais is designed to improve body awareness by focusing on sensory-motor learning itself, instead of strength or flexibility of muscles. The idea is to build flexible brains versus flexible bodies. The increased ability to make sensory distinctions enables the patient to experience new, pain-free patterns of whole body coordination. Movement dysfunction is caused, not by performing specific activities, but by doing them incorrectly. Therefore, movement reeducation for the body and mind is considered to be the most effective way to alleviate stress and pain.

In treatment sessions, the instructor guides the patient in activities which convey comfort and ease of movement; the patient learns to recognize the accompanying sensations and to internalize and recreate them. New patterns of movement are learned which are designed to expand body awareness and improve body image. In addition to improved movement, Feldenkrais is said to improve an individual's overall thinking ability and self-awareness through the increased capacity to make distinctions.

Feldenkrais uses two different techniques. "Awareness through Movement" provides group lessons of highly structured movement explorations. "Functional Integration" provides one-to-one, hands on therapy, until a patient can direct his own movements. In cases of neurologic or orthopedic disorders, the latter is used. The Feldenkrais Method is usually administered by physical or occupational therapists who have taken courses in this approach's clinical application.[10,11,12,13]

Alexander Technique

"A subjective sense of kinesthetic lightness is the Alexander Technique's hallmark." Frank Pierce Jones[4]

The Alexander Technique is a mind-body approach which teaches conscious control over body posture and movement for a better overall use of oneself. The three aspects of the approach are to use the whole back correctly, deal efficiently with gravity and eliminate muscle tension.[1] By using the back properly, one moves with less tension and fatigue and with greater ease; moving this way increases the injured body's ability to heal itself. All back conditions can be made better or worse by the way the head, neck and back are aligned and balanced during daily activities.

The four "concepts of good use" involve releasing the muscles so that they work only as much as they need to for a particular task.

1) allow the neck to release so that the head can balance forward and up
2) allow the torso to release into length and width
3) allow the legs to release away from the pelvis
4) allow the shoulders to release out to the sides.

In the initial session the instructor changes the posture of a patient's head to establish a new dynamic balance between the weight of the head and

127

response of the muscles; this allows the head to move freely without a feeling of weight. Then the same balance is achieved while performing activities. In later sessions this dynamic balance is worked on for the other three "concepts of good use" and expanded to a variety of activities. The overall goal is for patients to eliminate old, stereotyped responses and achieve a better, freer use of body and mind. Patients report feeling lighter and moving more easily.[1,4]

To become instructors in the Alexander Technique, individuals must complete 1600 hours of training over a minimum three-year period.

Synopses of
Other Movement Reeducation Approaches

"Can it be summed up so?" Robert Bridges
"I will not let thee go"

Aston-Patterning
Aston-Patterning, originally developed with Ida Rolf, is a system that integrates movement education, three different forms of soft tissue mobilization, environmental modification and fitness training. An evaluation determines the restrictions limiting movement options; treatment aims at facilitating change throughout the body to create an environment where abnormal or restricted movement doesn't have to occur. Instead of tensing the muscles to hold a new alignment, the patient performs exercises which loosen patterns of tension for a more restful relationship of body parts. The patient experiences change, learns how to facilitate that change independently and to then apply it to functional activities.[7]

Aikido
Aikido, or "The Way of Harmony with the Universe," is an Eastern-based mind-body discipline. It is used with pain patients to help them develop the inner resources to learn new movements and escape the restrictions that limit their options and keep them in pain. The practitioner seeks to blend with the patient's inherent unconscious movements and achieve a rapport or shared energy that allows the patient to experience changed movement patterns.[9]

Hellerwork
Hellerwork is based on the work of Joseph Heller, who was originally

trained in Rolfing. Heller's approach emphasizes structural balance and movement education; it incorporates deep tissue massage, releasing fascial restrictions, postural alignment and body awareness. Hellerwork also addresses emotional stress which creates tension patterns in posture and movement. Its goal is to realign the body and release chronic tension and stress; Hellerwork practitioners do not claim to treat medical problems.[3]

NDT
Neurodevelopmental Treatment was developed in England by Karl and Berta Bobath; it was originally used in the treatment of children with cerebral palsy. NDT emphasizes the normalization of muscle tone, such as inhibiting hypertonus and balancing flexor/extensor tone. This is followed by facilitation of the normal components of moving and weight-bearing. The goal is for stability against gravity with simultaneous functional mobility.[14] NDT principles are now used in the treatment of a variety of disabilities, including back pain.

PNF
Proprioceptive Neuromuscular Facilitation is an approach which promotes total movement patterns; the goal is to encourage motor learning. The name of this approach literally means hastening the response of the nervous and muscular systems through stimulation of the sensory receptors located in the tissues of the body. PNF is based on the belief that recapitulation of the sequence of human developmental milestones has value for all patients. Stronger parts of the body are utilized to stimulate and strengthen weaker parts; their cooperation leads to optimal function.[5]

Trager Therapy
Trager Therapy, or Psychophysical Integration, utilizes movement to produce positive, pleasurable sensory feelings. These enter the central nervous system and facilitate pain-free movement by means of the many sensory-motor feedback loops between the mind and the muscles.[10]

Key Points - Movement Reeducation

Treatment approaches which incorporate movement reeducation include Rolfing, the Feldenkrais Method, the Alexander Technique, Hellerwork and more. They share an emphasis on facilitating a new awareness of body movement and proper body alignment. Stress and structural imbalance restrict and alter movement; treatment removes the restrictions, releases tension and allows new and better movement patterns to be learned. The goal is a more comfortable, efficient and freer use of body and mind.

Footnotes

1   Deborah Caplan, *Back Trouble*
2   Brian Fahey, "The Principles of Structural Diagnosis"
3   Heller & Hanson, *The Client's Handbook*
4   Frank Pierce Jones, *Body Awareness in Action: A Study of the Alexander Technique*
5   Knott & Voss, *Proprioceptive Neuromuscular Facilitation*
6   Jason Mixter, "Rolfing"
7   Nancy Richardson, "Aston-Patterning"
8   Ida Rolf, "Structural Integration"
9   Gary Shapiro, "Ceasing the Struggle"
10 Weiselfish & Kain, "Introduction of Developmental Manual Therapy"
11 Frank Wildman, "The Feldenkrais Method: Clinical Applications"
12 Frank Wildman, "Learning - The Missing Link in Physical Therapy"
13 Frank Wildman, "Training in the Feldenkrais Method"
14 Julie Zimmerman, *Goals and Objectives for Developing Normal Movement Patterns*

Chapter 15 - "Point Therapy"

"Science moves, but slowly, slowly, creeping on from point to point." Lord Alfred Tennyson, "Locksley Hall"

The treatment approaches discussed in this chapter are concerned with acupuncture points, trigger points and reflex points; for that reason they have been grouped under the heading "point therapy."

Acupuncture

"O, be drest; Stay not for th' other pin!" George Herbert, "The Temple"

This 5000-year-old system of medicine is based on the theory of vital energy the Chinese call Qi (pronounced chee). Qi is the life force that circulates through the body and its balance is considered to be the essence of health. A balanced flow of Qi insures harmony between the two conflicting influences on the body, Yin and Yang. Yin connotes softness, darkness, coldness and wetness, while Yang connotes hardness, brightness, heat and dryness; various diseases can be explained by an excess or deficiency of one relative to the other. Health is maintained when Yin and Yang are in balance and Qi flows uninterrupted. Meridians are the 12 channels of vital energy which extend throughout the body, each associated with a different body system, but all interconnected. The connection between the meridians insures an even circulation of Qi which insures a balance of Yin and Yang. There are hundreds of points on the skin where meridians emerge on the surface.

Pain or illness, including back problems, results when the body's energy flow is disrupted or blocked or when Yin or Yang becomes excessive or deficient. An acupuncturist can ascertain, through the exact location of symptoms, which meridian and body system are involved. Acupuncture points on the skin are the endpoints of the meridians and stimulating these points can affect the flow of Qi. The insertion of needles can keep the energy system open and restore balance between Yin and Yang by strengthening Yin while eliminating excess Yang or vice versa. Specific results claimed by acupuncture include the following.[4,6,9,11]

- increased ability to fight disease
- improved hormonal functioning
- regeneration of nerve fibers
- lowered fevers
- restoration of gasto-intestinal function
- pain reduction through the production of endorphins (the body's own pain-killers).

Western medicine also uses acupuncture as a treatment for pain, but with a different rationale. The sensory stimulation produced by acupuncture is thought to produce a sharp decrease in back pain through "pain inhibition." Pain is blocked because the messages from nerves which carry pain impulses are inhibited by faster moving impulses from sensory nerves. This is called "gate control theory". [See Box 15-1]

> ## Gate Control Theory
>
> Normally, cells in the spinal cord act as censors, moderating the flow of sensory information from the body to the brain. According to gate control theory, impulses from sensory nerves travel faster than pain impulses and "close the gate" so that the slower pain messages do not get to the brain. When a sudden unpleasant stimulus crosses the pain threshold, the gate opens, allowing the sensation to spill over into consciousness.[5,7] Any stimulation that activates sensory nerves, such as rubbing the skin, affects pain perception. When someone bangs his head or raps his shin, he commonly rubs where it hurts; the injury itself is not reduced, but it feels better because rubbing the skin inhibits the pain.
>
> The opposite effect occurs when reduced sensory input increases pain perception. People are normally more aware of any kind of pain at rest; this is because at rest there is decreased visual, joint, muscle and skin stimulation.[7] To use gate control theory to help back pain patients, the goal is for maximum stimulation of sensory nerves with minimum pain stimulation.[5] Since people with back problems spend more time resting, one method for inhibiting pain is to gradually increase their activity levels.
>
> ### Box 15-1

With acupuncture, small needles are inserted into the surface of the skin at selected points; these acupuncture points have a smaller amount of electrical resistance than that of surrounding skin. The needles remain in place for about 20 minutes. Small clips which conduct heat or electricity from a machine are sometimes attached to the ends of the needles; this provides additional kinds of sensory stimulation.

Shiatzu

"If you want to be free of low back pain, welcome to Shiatzu!" Yukiko Irwin[4]

Shiatzu is the art of Japanese finger pressure. Thumb and finger pressure is used on acupuncture points to reduce pain caused by tension or muscle strain. It is not recommended for severe or chronic problems, such as disk rupture or degenerative disease. Acupuncture points are seen as the floodgates which keep the body's energy system open; when blocked energy results in poor health, pressure on these points restores a balanced flow. Shiatzu is thought to result in muscle relaxation, elimination of tension and increased blood flow. It is most often used to maintain health, whereas acupuncture is used to treat disease.[4]

Meridian Therapy

"About 40 percent of patients treated with Meridian Therapy remained free of complaints a year after therapy." Jan Dommerholt[3]

Meridian Therapy was developed by Christel Heidemann and based on three concepts. These are . . .
- connective tissue massage
- Taoist philosophy, (man is a component of the cosmic harmony)
- Anthroposophical Medicine, (pathology is a disturbance of the balanced relationship between the four stages of man - physical, ether, astral and spiritual).

In Meridian Therapy, colors are used to correct imbalances which occur in the meridians, or channels which carry the vital energy of the body. Every meridian responds to two specific colors; one stimulates and one decreases the energy flow. In treatment, bits of colored silk are taped to spots on the meridians with the goal of normalizing energy flow.[3]

Trigger Point Therapy

"Myofascial trigger points are an extremely common and, for those professionals who have learned to identify and manage them, an eminently treatable source of low back pain." David Simons, MD, and Janet Travell, MD[10]

An acute strain from overload or overstretch to muscles can initiate "myofascial trigger points"; these are self-sustaining, hyperirritable spots which are located in muscles or fascia. They are perpetuated by a variety of orthopedic or systemic conditions; these include chronic strain, a short leg, recurrent infections, metabolic disorders, uncontrolled allergies, emotional stress and many others. Trigger points are thought by some to be located on meridians.[1]

An active trigger point causes a variety of musculoskeletal complaints.
- referred pain
- decreased joint range of motion
- decreased muscle strength
- a twitch response upon stimulation of the muscle
- shortened palpable bands of taut fibers within the muscle
- spots of deep tenderness within the muscle.

Treatment aims at deactivating trigger points to achieve restoration of full muscle length and strength; sustained relief also requires resolution of the factors which activated the trigger points. Three treatment techniques used are . . .

1) passive stretch of the muscle during application of a vapocoolant spray which inhibits pain and spasm

2) precise injection of the trigger point with an anesthetic agent (procaine hydrochloride, .5 percent in saline)

3) ischemic compression of trigger points (manual pressure deep enough to block circulation to the site).

When a patient's site of pathology is too painful to treat directly, trigger points can be treated as an interim measure to reduce pain indirectly.[1,10]

Myotherapy for Trigger Points

"Most people don't have to suffer pain. Most pain can be erased by what you are about to learn." Bonnie Prudden[8]

"Myotherapy" is a treatment approach with a different concept of trigger points than that in "trigger point therapy." It is theorized that these highly irritable spots are laid down in muscle tissue throughout life by any insult, such as birth trauma, accidents, sports or occupational stresses or injuries, diseases or emotional stress. They can lie quiet in muscles for years, then in the right circumstances, become activated, causing the muscle to go into spasm. The spasm can be treated by a variety of methods, but the trigger point remains to flare up again later. If severe, it can lay down satellite trigger points in other muscles.

Myotherapy is specifically directed at eliminating trigger points. About seven seconds of deep pressure is exerted directly on the trigger point, denying oxygen to the area. The most common cause of back pain, according to myotherapists, is poorly conditioned musculature sent into spasm by

135

trigger points. Treatment with exercise, conditioning and myotherapy is said to be 95 percent effective.[8]

Foot Reflexology

"Reflexology will free you from sickness and suffering and fear of pain, when used correctly." Mildred Carter[2]

The author of a book on foot reflexology claims, *"This book shows you how easily it is possible to activate natural and prompt relief from practically all your aches and pains."* [2] The basis of foot reflexology is that various body parts are connected with certain reflex areas on the bottoms of the feet; sore spots on the feet represent sluggish, diseased parts of the body. Massaging these reflex buttons has a direct effect on specific body parts, sending a surge of stimulation to clear out the congestion and restore health. Reflexology is said to send an invigorating flow of circulation to every part of the body, providing almost immediate relief from pain and, in many cases, complete healing.

The spine is represented from the big toe to the heel along the inside of the foot. Foot reflexology is used for individuals with back problems to relieve malalignments and impinged nerves which cause tension, ("the cause of a big majority of our ailments").[2] Treatment aims to relax tension by allowing blood to flow freely, washing away poisons. With tension erased, muscles cease to contract, nerve impingements are relieved and vertebrae can return to their normal position.

Reflexology also treats the tension which is created by negative feelings, such as fear, anger and sadness. In addition to leading stressful lives, people in modern society no longer walk barefooted, like early man; going barefoot and using foot reflexology are recommended to stimulate the feet, keeping all parts healthy.[2]

Key Points - "Point Therapy"

Acupuncture, Shiatzu, Meridian Therapy and Foot Reflexology are all concerned with restoring a balanced flow of energy to an unhealthy body. Pain and illness are thought to result when energy flow is disrupted; treatment is carried out by stimulating specific points on the skin. Another view of acupuncture is that it works by blocking the transmission of pain messages through the use of sensory stimulation. Trigger point therapy and myotherapy direct treatment at specific sites within the muscles, called trigger points. Deactivation of trigger points reduces muscle pain and restriction.

Footnotes

1 "Approaches to Musculoskeletal Problems: Focus on the Low Back" Symposium, Kristian Arnold

2 Mildred Carter, *Helping Yourself with Foot Reflexology*

3 Jan Dommerholt, "Meridian Therapy - A New European Concept"

4 Yukiko Irwin, *Shiatzu*

5 David Lamb, "The Neurology of Spinal Pain"

6 Mills & Finando, *Alternatives in Healing*

7 Stanley Paris, *The Spine*

8 Bonnie Prudden, *Pain Erasure*

9 Carolyn Reuben, "AIDS: The Promise of Alternative Treatments"

10 Simons & Travell, "Myofascial Origins of Low Back Pain"

11 Wallnofer & vonRottauscher, *Chinese Folk Medicine and Acupuncture*

Chapter 16 - Oral Treatment

"The stomach - in its own particular method, it deals with the nourishment offered by the universe." Charles Williams

There is an increasing emphasis among alternative health practitioners on the profound connection between good nutrition and a healthy, injury-free body.[1] However, the claim that various diets, vitamins or natural potions provide relief from all health problems is an obvious oversimplification. Consumer Reports states that most Americans get at least enough nutrients from their diets. *"It is a distorted notion that many diseases are caused from poor nutrition and can be cured with large doses of vitamins or special diets."*[3] As with so many other treatment approaches to back pain, the patient should consider diet as only one factor in an overall health plan.

Diet

"50 percent of spinal pain can result from red meats." Bernice Krumhansl, PT, and Charles Nowacek, MD[6]

An improper diet and lifestyle is thought by some to be the root of most of our medical problems, while a natural foods diet based on whole grains and vegetables is the necessary foundation of health and well-being.[5] The theory is that poor eating habits weaken the entire fabric of the body's tissues. Nutritional food, on the other hand, has the ability to support and stimulate the immune system and is a safe, effective way to stay well. The goal of a healthy diet is to rebalance the body and promote self-healing.[1,2]

Four theories of the effects of diet on low back pain follow.

1) Excessive calcium in the diet can lead to bone spurs; eliminating meat and milk allows a disturbed calcium mechanism to readjust. One "macrobiotic" diet prohibits meat, milk and nightshades (potatoes, tomatoes, tobacco); success has been reported with macrobiotics in restoring joint flexibility and shrinking bone spurs. Eliminating nightshades and vitamin D has also been known to alleviate low back pain.[2]

2) Red meat, and to a lesser extent fish and fowl, cause muscles to swell, shorten and become sluggish; the result is stiffness and limitation, especially in the mid to low spine.[6]

3) Changes in body chemistry from the wrong diet irritates the gall bladder and liver, causing an excessively acidic condition. This, in turn, irritates the nerves, causing pain anywhere in the body.[6]

4) Nutrition can influence the meninges, which cover the brain and spinal cord. Excess fat in the diet causes a distortion in the way energy is used and impedes its smooth flow through the meninges and cerebro-spinal fluid. Mechanical problems of the spinal column are the end result.[7] (The role of the meninges in maintaining health is discussed in Chapter 13, "Fascia Based Treatments.")

Many see dietary changes as only one aspect of overall improvement in lifestyle. *"Most cures as an apparent result of diet have included a profound life change on the emotional-spiritual level; with serious illness the best diet is only minimally effective without that inner change."*[2] Some theorize a link between certain foods and spiritual, societal views. For example, the high consumption of nightshades is associated with intellectual activity and materialism as well as with the increase of health problems in our mechanized society.[2]

Vitamins

"Oranges and lemons, Say the bells of St. Clement's." Tommy Thumb's Pretty Song Book
c. 1744

Massive doses of certain vitamins are consumed for a variety of health problems. Vitamin C has been advocated for people with rheumatic conditions, who tend to have low levels of Vitamin C in the blood. It has also been used for people taking aspirin, as aspirin is thought to interfere with the retention of Vitamin C in the body.[4] Chiropractors, among others, advocate the use of vitamins, but many consider this a health risk; taking large doses of vitamins can cause serious side effects, in the same way prescription medications can.[3]

Herbalism

"Tis healthy to be sick sometimes." Henry David Thoreau

Holistic healers may use medications, but only those found in nature; their emphasis remains on allowing the body to heal itself. Medical herbalism is a treatment approach which uses medications exclusively from plant materials, specifically extracts from the whole plant versus isolated ingredients which can prove harmful. Herbalism is concerned with the individual nature of the patient, not just in treating separately defined illnesses. Disease is seen as a result of the body's own attempt to restore balance and harmony; treatment is aimed at supporting rather than suppressing the body's healing mechanisms.[8] (See *, paragraph 2 under Homeopathy, for the application of herbalism to back pain.)

Homeopathy

"Aggravation of symptoms is part of the healing process." Simon Mills and Steven Finando, PhD[8]

Homeopathy regards the symptoms of an illness as expressions of disharmony in the body. It bases treatment on the concept of "like cures like," with medications mimicking the symptoms of a disease. The first reaction of such treatment is to worsen the symptoms, but as symptoms are the expression of the body fighting disease, the ultimate result is to hasten healing. Disease is seen as the combination of symptoms produced by the body in its own effort to heal itself. If symptoms are suppressed, disease is prolonged.[8]

*The role of herbalism and homeopathy in the treatment of back pain doesn't follow the "like cures like" principle; pain is apparently not considered a natural symptom of the self-healing process. *"There are some cases that a homeopath would prefer not to tackle and backache is one of them."*[8] For back problems, herbs or medications might be prescribed to ...

- alleviate pain
- improve muscle tone
- remove toxins from joints or muscles
- correct vitamin deficiency
- reduce muscle tension
- improve circulation
- promote relaxation
- reduce stress.

For conditions such as ruptured disks or degenerative disease of the spine, recommendations from a homeopath or herbalist would include a referral for osteopathic or chiropractic manipulation, Alexander Technique training, etc.[8]

Key Points - Oral Treatment

Theories have been proposed that many diseases are the result of poor nutrition and can be cured with special diets or large doses of vitamins. Certain diets have been specifically recommended for people with back pain. Herbalism and homeopathy are approaches which treat disease with medications which support the body's healing mechanisms versus suppressing symptoms of the disease. The possible effects of diet and natural medications on back pain are discussed in this chapter. Patients should be aware that there are risks connected with excessive use of oral substances, even those found in nature.

Footnotes

1 Ben Benjamin, "The Mystery of Lower Back Pain"
2 Annemarie Colbin, *Food and Healing*
3 Consumer Reports Books, *Health Quackery*
4 Norman Cousins, *Anatomy of an Illness*
5 Ronald Kotzch, "AIDS: Putting an Alternative to the Test"
6 Krumhansl & Nowacek, "Case Study - Spinal Manipulation Under Anaesthesia"
7 Mark Mead, "Chiropractic's New Wave"
8 Mills & Finando, *Alternatives in Healing*

Chapter 17 - Mind/Spirit Approaches

"Society seems to think if you eat right, think right and jog you should never be sick, so if you are it's your fault." Betsy Lehman[7]

Researchers are deeply divided on the connection between attitude and disease. *"Twenty years ago hardly anyone thought mind and body were related, but we have now swung to a belief just as simplistic and inaccurate that illness is created in the mind."*[7] The new emphasis on personal responsibility can empower patients, but can also place an unfair burden on people with health problems. A positive outlook does help some patients feel better and certainly improves the quality of life, but it is not the cure for everyone's back pain. It is unfair for advocates of this approach to believe that their successes validate their theories, while their failures are the responsibility of the patient.

The approaches covered in this chapter concern people's use of their spiritual, mental and emotional strength and energy to improve their health.

The discussions focus on four of the most well-known writers in the area of healing through the power of the mind and spirit. However, every practitioner has his or her own unique philosophy which may not coincide with that of the "experts". Furthermore, individuals can draw on their own inner resources to direct positive energy toward the relief of back pain.

Mind Over Back Pain

"I believe my TMS patients cure themselves once I have provided them with the proper information." John Sarno, MD[9]

John Sarno has coined the phrase Tension Myositis Syndrome (TMS) to describe what he considers to be the primary cause of back pain. TMS is a harmless disorder of the muscles and nerves caused by reduced blood flow to these tissues. Circulation is constricted due to tension, especially common in certain personality types. He explains that injuries or structural abnormalities of the spine are rarely responsible for common backache; "the spine is perfectly sound; the culprit is excessive tension in an age of anxiety."[9] Sarno believes that conventional diagnoses, such as degenerative disk disease or arthritis, contribute to the severity and persistence of pain; they frighten patients and increase tension. Conventional treatments, (bedrest, mechanical supports, postural restrictions), send the message that the condition is more serious than it is, further increasing tension. Since pain is caused by TMS, most treatments, (manipulation, back exercises, acupuncture, biofeedback, surgery), are not effective, work only temporarily or succeed only because of the placebo effect.[9]

If TMS were explained to patients, they would know the process is self-limiting; instead of fear leading to increased pain, they would feel reassured, setting in motion a positive cycle. Sarno believes that patients should be taught to think of pain in psychological terms so it is no longer expressed physically. Once the patient realizes the pain is due to tension and not structural abnormalities, the pain stops. The knowledge results in a permanent cure because it prevents the nervous system from transmitting nerve impulses that constrict blood vessels. Patients who accept the idea of TMS improve; those who reject the idea don't.[9]

Sarno tends to attribute successful outcomes from other treatment to the placebo effect. One patient received significant help from reading Sarno's book for a low back condition; however, despite his enthusiasm for the approach, it provided no relief for a later neck problem. Writing about those experiences later, he states, *"Sarno quotes great cure rates in his book and points out that his failures are usually people who refuse to accept the diagnosis. I had a terrible thought: What if those people were right?"*[1]

Laughter

"Wrinkles should merely indicate where smiles have been." Mark Twain

Norman Cousins is well known for his books on the importance of positive thought and laughter in the treatment of illness. He believes that emotions such as love, faith, confidence, hope and the will to live mobilize the body's natural mechanisms to fight disease. The patient's faith in the effectiveness of the treatment has a major role in bringing about a cure. Doctors are advised to encourage an optimistic outlook in their patients in order to use all the resources of body and mind. Cousins advocates a partnership between physician and patient, with the patient taking as much responsibility as possible for selecting a treatment and participating in its application.[2]

Some studies show that humor relieves pain and other symptoms, although the disease itself is still present; laughter can stimulate the production of endorphins, the body's own pain-killers.[3] It is also theorized that laughter may reduce the risk of developing health problems, slow their progression or that it can actually cure.[8] Another theory is that laughing or assuming a happy facial expression may induce a positive mood, rather than vice versa. What is certain is that humor improves the quality of anyone's life.

Critics of Cousins' writings are concerned that he overemphasizes the shortcomings of the medical field and exaggerates the value of supportive methods.[4] *"Humor tries to make light of death and disability. When the context is the constructive acceptance of reality, that's good. It's not good, however, if humor is used to promote a therapeutic environment in which we are encouraged to abandon rationality, to trust anecdote, to embrace anti-science."*[4]

Chapter 17

Spiritual Healing
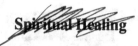

Spiritual or metaphysical healers, such as Louise Hay, believe that reality is a construct of the mind; therefore illness is also created by the mind and manifested in the body. Negative beliefs and emotions create trauma which becomes registered in tissues as blocked energy. In spiritual healing, patients are helped to recall the trauma and connect it to a specific symptom. The negative feelings are then replaced with affirmations of positive truth and forgiveness.

Louise Hay feels that we are each 100 percent responsible for all of our experiences, including the creation of every "so-called" physical illness.[6] Everyone suffers from self-hatred and guilt and such negative mental patters create disease in the body. Hay equates very specific negative feelings to very specific symptoms.[6]

- Chronic pain is caused by chronic guilt.
- Back problems in general are due to a lack of feeling supported.
- Low back pain is due to financial worries.
- Mid back pain is due to guilt.
- Upper back pain is due to a lack of emotional support.
- Neck pain is caused by being stubborn and inflexible.'

In treatment, Hay works on loving oneself, using affirmations, guided imagery and meditation to change negative mental patterns and allow healing. Therapies such as acupuncture, Rolfing, deep massage and Shiatzu may also be used with spiritual healing to stimulate energy flow through the body parts where negative feelings are stored.

Crystals are used by some healers to help dislodge inhibitions which block the flow of higher life energies. Crystal pieces are placed on the body where there is pain or held near the source of pain. It is said that they amplify the positive energy from the healer and focus it on the patient for healing. Crystals are also through to draw out the problem which is causing the pain, allowing a rebalancing of the body's energy.[5]

Spiritual healers make a point of differentiating responsibility from blame. However, many tend to believe that if treatment is unsuccessful, it is because the patient is unwilling to take responsibility for his or her illness. Since all illness is supposedly based in spiritual negativity, an unsuccessful outcome to treatment can create significant guilt and stress in a patient.

Positive Feelings

"I believe that all disease is ultimately related to a lack of love or to conditional love."
Bernie Siegel, MD[10]

Bernie Siegel's books and workshops concern the power of feelings to cause or cure disease. Feelings are closely connected to body chemistry, as demonstrated by the strength of the placebo effect; patients who think a treatment will help have been shown to produce endorphins, a natural pain-killer. Endorphins are only one of many substances known to be produced by the brain. Their effect demonstrates that what takes place in the body can be changed by changing the state of mind. By using processes that alter their feelings, people open themselves up to physical changes, including healing. Healing can be set in motion by self-affirming beliefs, while self-negating or repressive emotional patterns can do the reverse.[10]

The body is capable of manufacturing symptoms to meet one's needs; emotional or spiritual problems are eventually expressed physically. When emotional or physical needs are denied, the body's healing system is blocked and receives the message that recovery isn't desired; illness may serve the purpose of providing a way to get one's needs met. Patients are asked to play an active role in health care, sending positive mental images to the body to empower it to achieve what is visualized. Health practitioners have a responsibility to offer hope, in whatever treatment form, to give their patients the potential to heal themselves.[10] Techniques for achieving a positive state of mind include visualization, yoga, hypnosis, psychotherapy, mediation and relaxation training. (Some of these treatments were discussed in Chapter 7, "Relaxation Techniques".)

Siegel cites studies that suggest mental attitudes affect susceptibility to disease and the ability to overcome it; hopelessness and helplessness are found to be factors in developing ill health. What creates the best chance for self-healing and healthy bodies are the following:[10]
- a sense of meaning and purpose in life
- taking personal responsibility for one's health
- the ability to express needs and emotions

• a sense of humor.

Patients, however, are not demanded to get well. Even if the disease is not cured, the goal is for them to heal their lives. In other words, the success is not in length of life, but in its quality.[10]

Bernie Siegel's theory on the relation between feelings and disease have created significant controversy. The conflict is centered on one question he asks patients to ask themselves, *"Why do you need your illness and what benefits do you derive from it?"* Siegel emphasizes that he is not blaming patients for their illnesses and that continuing dysfunction should not cause guilt. The fact is, however, that blame and guilt is what some readers take from his approach.

Siegel's books are popular and many people have found them inspiring; however, people in pain are emotionally vulnerable and may be quick to feel pressured or guilty. Friends and relatives of people with newly diagnosed or chronic illnesses may want to think twice before giving these books as gifts; the giver may be sending an unintentional message. A woman newly diagnosed with cancer commented, "I was given three copies of his book and I hated them all."

Key Points - Mind/Spirit Approaches

There is much controversy concerning the connection between attitude and disease. This chapter includes the theories of John Sarno, Norman Cousins, Louise Hay and Bernie Seigel. All stress the importance of a positive attitude and participation of the patient in curing the illness; a belief in the philosophy of the healer also seems to be a requirement. Emphasizing personal responsibility can empower a patient and a positive attitude improves the quality of life. However, these approaches may place an unfair burden on people with health problems; too often the patient is held responsible for continuing symptoms and is left feeling guilty and isolated.

Footnotes

1   Henry Allen, "That Back's Gotta Come Out"

2   Norman Cousins, *Anatomy of an Illness*

3   Pat Croce, "Put Stress to Rest"

4   Neil Elgee, "Norman Cousins' Sick Laughter Redux"

5   Phyllis Glade, *Crystal Healing: The Next Step*

6   Louise Hay, *You Can Heal Your Life*

7   Betsy Lehman, "Feeling Bad About Feeling Bad"

8   P.T. Bulletin, "Benefits of 'Humor Therapy' Promoted"

9   John Sarno, *Mind Over Back Pain*

10 Bernie Siegel, *Peace, Love and Healing*

Chapter 18 - Author's Recommendations

". . .advice is a dangerous gift, even from the wise to the wise, and all courses may run ill."
J.R.R. Tolkien, *The Fellowship of the Ring*

Comments Concerning Diagnosis and Treatment

The approaches discussed in *The Almanac of Back Pain Treatments* have critics as well as avid proponents. This reinforces the fact that every treatment for back pain helps some patients, but not one can help every patient. The premise of this book reflects the confusion and controversy surrounding this condition; it is that **the diagnosis and treatment of back pain must be individualized.**

Unfortunately, many people assume that "most" patients with back pain have the same problem and require the same type of intervention. The following diagnoses and treatments are appropriate and successful for some patients, but they are too often applied indiscriminately. Practitioners who are too committed to a philosophy tend to blame the patient if the treatment is unsuccessful. [See Box 18-1]

One-Size-Fits-All Approaches to Back Pain

Diagnosis	Practitioner	Treatment
somatic dysfunction	osteopath	manipulation
vertebral subluxation	chiropractor	spinal adjustment
back strain	MD	bedrest, heat, medications, corset
arthritis	MD	symptomatic treatment
weak abdominals	any & all	flexion exercises
stress/tension	any & all	relaxation techniques, counseling

Practitioners of many alternative approaches, (spiritual healing, Rolfing, myotherapy, foot reflexology, myofascial release, craniosacral therapy, Feldenkrais, Alexander Technique, Tension Myositis Syndrome treatment, acupuncture and macrobiotics), may regard all back pain as the result of a single factor. These presumed causes include blocked energy, fascial restrictions, unresolved emotions, tension, poor nutrition or negative feelings.

Box 18-1

Health professionals with expertise in tailoring exercises to the individual back pain patient include physiatrists (MDs specializing in rehabilitation and physical medicine), physical therapists and sports medicine doctors. Other practitioners who can individualize exercise programs include kinesiologists (experts in the principles and mechanics of movement), and Yoga or physical fitness instructors with special training in back dysfunction.[2]

Recommendations for People with Back Pain

Despite variation and controversy in the treatment of back pain, there are some general guidelines which can be applied to every back problem. The following recommendations are meant for anyone with back pain; like all advice, apply it judiciously to your own situation.

1) Find a health care professional with whom you can communicate and work together to understand and treat your back pain. Ask about the rationale of various treatments in order to avoid having unrealistic expectations.

2) Keep bedrest to a minimum; a maximum of 2 days is now considered sufficient for most acute episodes. Alternate bedrest with a brief period of moving about every 1-2 hours.

3) Both performing pelvic tilts and the application of heat can be effective in relieving muscle spasm. However, during the first 24-48 hours following an episode of acute pain, try using ice instead of heat; it is considered preferable for the reduction of inflammation.

4) Minimize your use of medications, especially on a long-term basis.

5) Avoid surgery as a cure for pain; there are very clear and limited conditions for which surgery is appropriate.

6) There is evidence that vigorous manipulation has no advantage over mobilization techniques; the gentlest kind of manual therapy which is effective is recommended. If manipulation is the appropriate treatment for your condition, there should be significant improvement in pain or mobility within 3 treatments.

7) Whether on bedrest, working, driving or relaxing, change position frequently. Immobility is bad for backs.

8) If you were injured on the job, a rehabilitation program that simulates your work place can speed your return to work; discuss a referral to a "Work Hardening" program with your doctor.

9) A back condition requires the right balance of rest, activity and common sense. Listen to your body; society may place a premium on being tough, but a "no pain, no gain" approach is overrated.

10) Consider the role of stress or tension in your back pain and don't be afraid to incorporate relaxation techniques or counseling as one component of your overall treatment program. However, if your practitioner automatically assumes your pain is emotionally based and you disagree, feel free to seek a second opinion.

11) Without question, a positive attitude and sense of humor improve the quality of your life; they may do much more. However, they are unable to cure everyone's back pain. If a treatment approach is unsuccessful, don't assume it's because you didn't try hard enough.

12) There are few approaches without critics, but the following seem to be universally recommended. For pain reduction as well as prevention they should be incorporated into your daily routine for the rest of your life.
- good posture and body mechanics
- a physical conditioning program suited to your level of functioning

- attention to your overall health needs
- taking responsibility for the management of your back pain

If you're recovering from your first acute episode of back pain, you are probably horrified at the thought of repeating the experience. If your back pain is recurrent, you can't imagine living with it all the time. And yet once the pain goes, there is a tendency to return to old habits. A recent study in the *The New England Journal of Medicine* compared patients on an exercise program with a group that didn't exercise. The exercisers had significant improvement in both pain reduction and activity level. However, two months later *"most patients had discontinued the exercises and the initial improvements were gone."*[1] If you are fortunate enough to achieve pain relief by changing your lifestyle, make those changes permanent.

Recommended Reading

Lauren Hebert, *Sex and Back Pain* (a practical guide for finding comfortable positions for sex)

Barbara Headley, *Chronic Pain: Life Out of Balance* (an easy to read booklet on chronic pain issues, with cartoon drawings)

Klein & Sobel, *Backache Relief* (the results of a large survey of back pain patients)

Robin McKenzie, *Treat Your Own Back* (a guide to causes of back pain and specific exercise programs)

Melnick, Saunders & Saunders, *Managing Back Pain* (an easy to understand explanation of the effects of posture on the back, with recommended exercises)

Sefra Pitzele, *We Are Not Alone* (a book that explores the difficulties of living with chronic illness and offers practical help)

Cheri Register, *Living With Chronic Illness* (another personal view of chronic illness. Both Pitzele and Register are very helpful from an emotional standpoint.)

Duane Saunders, *The Back Care Program* (a practical and inexpensive guide for proper posture in all kinds of activities - a must!)

Duane Saunders, *For Your Neck* (a booklet on the effects of posture on neck pain, with recommended exercises)

Julie Zimmerman, *The Diagnosis and Misdiagnosis of Back Pain* (an in depth examination of the processes used to diagnose back pain, the approaches of different health professionals and the conditions which cause back pain)

Julie Zimmerman, *Chronic Back Pain: Moving On* (an examination of the causes and effects of chronic pain and the range of treatment and management options for people living with chronic back problems)

Recommendations for Health Professionals

Back pain is often a difficult and frustrating condition to diagnose and treat. It is important to take the time to truly asses and evaluate your patient, relating symptoms to the patient's functional mobility and structural abnormalities. Apply the appropriate treatments based on your evaluation and then reevaluate to determine the patient's response to treatment. Health care practitioners who are irrevocably dedicated to one philosophy may not best serve the back pain patient. As one physical therapist writes, *"We cannot afford to be narrow-minded or isolated in our treatment procedures. As our people are varied, so too are their neuromusculoskeletal systems; we must treat them individually and thoroughly."*[3]

Patients need to be reassured that low back syndrome is not life-threatening and need the chance to ask questions and discuss their anxieties. Many don't know whether your treatment approach is symptomatic or curative; many assume that when their pain is reduced, the home program you recommended is no longer necessary. They need to understand that many of the most effective treatments for back pain require the patients to make permanent life-style changes, (e.g., posture, physical conditioning, exercise programs, common sense). It is in the interest of both practitioner and patient to work as a team, each with certain responsibilities. You don't have all the answers and should be able to admit that; the patient shouldn't expect to be given a magic bullet.

It is a major challenge to create an individualized program out of the broad range of treatment options available for back problems. Part of your arsenal in combatting your patient's back pain is the ability to make appropriate referrals; an awareness of your limitations is the mark of a fine and effective health professional.

Recommended Reading

Diagnosis
- Kirkaldy-Willis, "A More Precise Diagnosis for Low Back Pain"
- Paris, "Physical Signs of Instability"
- Headley, "Postural Homeostasis"

Physicians & Pain Patients
- Cassel, "The Nature of Suffering and the Goals of Medicine"
- Cailliet, *Low Back Pain Syndrome, 1988 edition*

Indications for Surgery
- Fager, "Beware the Quick Fix for Back Pain"
- Fager, "Facts and Fallacies of Spinal Disorders: A Neurosurgeon's Viewpoint"

Spondylosis
- Burkart & Beresford, "The Aging Intervertebral Disk"

Sacro-Iliac Joint Dysfunction
- Beal, "The Sacroiliac Problem: Review of Anatomy, Mechanics and Diagnosis"
- Bellamy, Park & Rooney, "What Do We Know About the Sacroiliac Joint"
- DonTigny, "Function and Pathomechanics of the Sacroiliac Joint"
- Grieve, "Lumbo-pelvic Rhythm and Mechanical Dysfunction of the Sacro-iliac Joint"

Exercise
- Jackson & Brown, "Analysis of Current Approaches and a Practical Guide to Prescription of Exercise"
- McGavin, "The McKenzie Approach to Spinal Pain"

Manipulation & Mobilization
- Consumer Reports Books, *Health Quackery*
- DiFabio, "Clinical Assessment of Manipulation and Mobilization of the Lumbar Spine"
- Paris, *The Spine* (course notes)

Overview of Musculoskeletal Dysfunction
- Kaplan & Tanner, *Musculoskeletal Pain and Disability*
- Kessler & Hertling, *Management of Common Musculoskeletal Disorders*
- Saunders, *Evaluation, Treatment and Prevention of Musculoskeletal Disorders*

Conclusion: Moving On

The Almanac of Back Pain Treatments is concerned with curing, relieving and managing acute, recurrent and chronic back pain. It attempts to give you, the back pain patient, enough information to understand the range of treatment possibilities available to you; it presents both their pros and cons. The goal is to allow you to make informed decisions to help in the difficult task of finding the answers that will minimize your back pain. When you have explored your options and followed through on your choices, then relegate the pain to a less central place in your life. It's time to return to the essential task of making the best of your world and yourself!

Footnotes

1   Richard Deyo, et al., "A Controlled Trial of Transcutaneous Electrical Nerve Stimulation (TENS) and Exercise for Chronic Low Back Pain"
2   Klein & Sobel, *Backache Relief*
3   David Reese, "Keep P.T. the Art That It Is"

Appendix A

Glossary

abduction - movement away from the midline of the body

active - performed through the effort of muscle contraction following nerve stimulation

acupressure - treatment approach using deep thumb or finger pressure on acupuncture points

acupuncture - treatment approach using needles inserted into the skin at points representing the body's meridians

acute - of recent onset; having a short, relatively severe course

acutherapy - acupuncture or acupressure

adduction - movement toward the midline of the body

adhesion - abnormal binding down of soft tissue

aerobics - exercise that increases the body's use of oxygen

ambulation - walking

ankylosing spondylitis - a form of arthritis, also called Marie Strumpel's disease

annulus fibrosis - the outer part of an intervertebral disk

anomaly - abnormality

antagonist - the muscle which performs movement in the opposite direction to the muscle being discussed

anterior - toward the front of the body

anterior dysfunction - displacement of the sacrum relative to the ilia, occurring on forward flexion

anterior superior iliac spine - bony landmark on the pelvis commonly called the "hip bone"

anterolateral - angled toward the front and side of the body

arachnoid - the middle of the three meninges

arthritis - a condition characterized by inflammation of the joints

articular - pertaining to a joint

articular cartilage - cartilaginous surface of a joint at the end of a bone

articular process - superior or inferior bony prominence of a vertebra which forms a facet joint with an adjacent vertebra

ASIS - see anterior superior iliac spine

asymptomatic - without symptoms; painless

atrophy - wasting or shrinking of muscle fibers

auto-immune - pertaining to conditions in which the body produces antibodies against its own tissues

autonomic nervous system - portion of the nervous system concerned with regulation of the heart muscle, smooth muscle and glands

back muscles - see spinal muscles

back school - a class offered by PT departments which teaches proper use of the spine

bedrest, total - bedrest during which any weight-bearing is eliminated or minimized

bilateral - involving both right and left sides of the body

biofeedback - a modality which visually or auditorally represents physiological responses of the body to enable patients to learn to consciously produce physical changes

body mechanics - the posture of the body in motion

bone - hard, immobile structure which makes up the skeleton or framework of the body

bone scan - radiographic test involving the injection of dye into a vein in order to identify diseases of bone

bone spur - abnormal growth of bony tissue often associated with degenerative changes

capsule - see joint capsule

cartilage - hard, structural tissue which makes up part of the skeleton; found at the ends of bones, ribs and joint surfaces

CAT scan - computerized axial tomography; a radiographic test which provides a three-dimensional picture of bone and soft tissue

catecholamines - compounds produced by the body in response to stress

cauda equina syndrome - a serious condition in which a nerve or nerves in the lower part of the spinal canal are compressed, causing bladder symptoms

central nervous system - the brain and spinal cord

cerebro-spinal fluid - a fluid produced by the brain which is contained between the meninges and which serves a shock-absorbing role for the central nervous system

cervical - pertaining to the neck region

cervical roll - cylindrical pillow placed behind the neck to maintain the cervical lordosis

chronic - long-lasting; pertaining to a medical condition lasting longer than three to six months

chronic pain syndrome - long-term pain which is reinforced by the environment and associated with a specific personality profile

coccyx - the vertebral segments comprising the tailbone

contract - shorten, referring to a muscle when stimulated

contraction - tensing or shortening of a muscle in response to a nerve stimulus

contraindicated - to be avoided; not recommended

contralateral - pertaining to the opposite side of the body

cortical bone - outer part of the shaft of a bone

cortisone - a hormone with anti-inflammatory properties

counterstrain - a technique which maintains the muscle in a relaxed, non-strained posture for 90 seconds

cranial - pertaining to the skull or head

craniosacral rhythm - the pulse produced by the cyclical production of CSF

CSF - see cerebro-spinal fluid

CT scan - see CAT scan

deafferation - the cutting of a sensory nerve

dermatome - skin area innervated by one spinal nerve

diathermy - machine which uses electricity to apply heat to surface tissues

differential diagnosis - the process of ruling out possible pathology to arrive at a definitive diagnosis

disc - see disk

disk - the structure located between the vertebral bodies, composed of a fibrous outer ring and an inner gelatin-like center

diskectomy - a surgical procedure to remove the disk or nucleus of the disk

disk fragment - extruded piece of the nucleus of the disk

diskography - a radiographic procedure in which dye is injected into a disk to identify a rupture

dislocation - total disruption of the opposing surfaces of a joint

DO - doctor of osteopathy

dural sheath (dura) - the outer covering of a nerve root

dura mater (dura) - the outermost of the three meninges which covers the brain and spinal cord
dysfunction - increased, decreased or abnormal movement

electromyography - diagnostic test in which needle electrodes inserted into muscle tissue relay
    electrical impulses from the muscle in order to identify nervous system diseases
electrotherapy - the therapeutic use of electricity
embryological - formed during the development of a fetus
EMG - see electromyography
endorphin - natural pain-killing substance produced by the body
endurance - lasting power; ability to maintain a position or perform numerous repetitions of a
    movement
ER - external rotation
erector spinae - back muscles which extend the trunk
ergonomics - adaptation of the workplace and equipment to accommodate an injured worker
extensibility - amount of stretch in a tissue
extension - motion of straightening a joint or body part
extensor muscles - see spinal muscles
external rotation - hip or shoulder movement in which the long bone of the thigh or arm rolls
    outward
extrusion - escaping of tissue outside its normal boundaries

facet joint - a synovial joint formed by the articular processes of two vertebrae
facilitation - see muscle facilitation
fascia - connective tissue of the body
femur - thigh bone
fiber - small segment of connective or muscle tissue; a nerve process
fibrillation - spontaneous contractions of individual muscle cells or fibers
fibromyalgia - see fibrositis
fibromyositis - see fibrositis
fibrositis - a condition characterized by diffuse tender areas of musculoskeletal tissues
flexion - motion of bending a joint or body part
function - use; movement
functional mobility - ability of the body to move normally to perform activities of daily living
functional restoration - work hardening
fusion - a surgical procedure in which bone fragments are inserted into an unstable joint to form
    a solid mass of bone

gate control theory - concept that pain sensations are blocked at the spinal cord by sensory
    stimulation
golfer's lift - stance incorporating extension of the non-weight bearing leg when bending forward
GP - general practitioner
gluteals - muscles at the back and sides of the pelvis which extend or abduct the hip
gluteal sets - tensing of the gluteus maximus muscles by squeezing the buttocks together

hamstrings - the muscles at the back of the thigh which extend the hip and flex the knee
herniated, herniation - see ruptured, rupture
holism - approach to health care which emphasizes the whole person
hyperextension - extension past a neutral trunk position
hypermobility - excessive movement of joints

161

hypomobility - below-average movement of joints
hypertonus - excessive amount of muscle tone

iatrogenic - caused by medical treatment
iliac crest - large curved portion of the upper pelvis, starting at what is commonly called the "hip bone"
ilium (pl. - ilia) - part of the pelvis which lies posterior and superior and forms a joint with the sacrum
impingement - compression, usually referring to a nerve root compression due to a disk rupture
inhibition - see muscle inhibition
innervation - nerve supply to a body part, usually referring to the nerve which stimulates a specific muscle
inominates - the joint surfaces of the pelvis which connect with the sacrum
internal rotation - a motion of the shoulder or hip joint in which the long bone of the upper arm or thigh rolls inward
interspinous ligaments - short ligaments connecting spinous processes of the vertebrae
intra-abdominal pressure - the tension of the contents of the abdomen against a contraction of the abdominal muscles
IR - internal rotation
internship - the year of hospital training following medical school
intervertebral - between the vertebrae
ischemia - decreased blood supply
ischium - part of the pelvis which lies posterior and inferior
isometrics - muscle contractions in which no joint movement occurs

joint - moveable part of the body's skeleton where the ends of two bones are joined
joint capsule - the sheath which surrounds and protects a synovial joint
joint play - small, involuntary movements in a joint in response to an outside force

kinesiology - the applied study of the principles and mechanics of movement
kinesiotherapy - a profession providing rehabilitation under the direction of physiatrist
KT - kinesiotherapist
kyphosis - convex curve of the spine, normal in the thoracic and sacral areas

lamina - the posterior part of the vertebral arch
laminectomy - surgical removal of the posterior arch of a vertebra, usually done to relieve nerve root compression from a ruptured disk
lateral flexion - movement of the neck or trunk to the side, away from the body's midline
lengthening contraction - tensing of a muscle to control movement in a direction opposite to its normal action
lesion - site of an injury
ligament - tough inelastic tissue which supports joints
longitudinal ligaments - long anterior and posterior ligaments running the length of the spinal column and connecting the vertebral bodies
long-sitting - sitting position with hips flexed and knees extended
lordosis - concave curve of the spine, normal in the cervical and lumbar areas
low back syndrome - vague diagnosis referring to non life-threatening conditions affecting the lumbo-sacral spine and its related structures
lumbago - common term for backache

lumbar - pertaining to the low back area

lumbar roll - approximately four-inch cylindrical pillow used to maintain a lumbar lordosis

magnetic resonance imaging - a non-invasive diagnostic test in which magnetic waves are used to image soft tissues

malingering - pretending to be ill

malleolus - ankle bone

manipulation - treatment approach in which the practitioner imparts a sudden thrust to realign body structures and/or reduce functional limitations

manual therapy - treatment in which the practitioner's hands are used to effect changes in the body

MD - medical doctor; one who has graduated from a four-year medical school

meninges - the three membranes which surround the brain and spinal cord

meniscus - crescent-shaped structure made up of cartilage and fibrous tissue which attaches to a joint capsule and extends into a joint

MENS - microcurrent therapy

meridian - one of 12 channels of vital energy in the body; a concept used in acupuncture

microcurrent therapy - form of electrotherapy which uses a current of low amperage to promote healing

mixers - chiropractors who use other treatment forms in addition to manipulation

mobilization - gentle form of manual therapy used to restore normal movement to body structures

MRI - magnetic resonance imaging

muscle - structure made up of elastic, contractile fibers which shortens when stimulated by a nerve to produce movement at a joint

muscle energy techniques - treatment which uses nervous system mechanisms to inhibit or facilitate a specific muscle

muscle facilitation - technique which uses nervous system mechanisms to increase muscle tone and stimulate a muscle to contract

muscle fatigue - technique using a strong contraction of a tight muscle to cause subsequent inhibition and relaxation of that muscle

muscle inhibition - use of nervous system mechanisms to reduce tone or spasm in tight muscles

muscle tone - see tone

myelogram - a radiographic test in which cerebro-spinal fluid is removed from the space surrounding the spinal cord and dye is injected in order to identify nerve root compression

myofascial - pertaining to the muscles and their surrounding connective tissue

myofascial pain syndrome - see fibrositis

nerve - a cell which transmits impulses within the nervous system to carry information to and from the brain or spinal cord; a bundle of nerve projections and their coverings

nerve root - part of the nervous system connecting the spinal cord and peripheral nerves which lies within the spinal canal

nerve root compression - pressure against a nerve root, commonly from a ruptured disk or bone spur, which produces pain and neurologic signs

neurological - neurologic

neurologic signs - symptoms which indicate involvement of the nervous system; with nerve root compression, numbness, weakness, decreased reflexes

neurology - a medical specialty which treats diseases of the nervous system

neurosurgery - a medical specialty where operations are performed on the nervous system or its surrounding structures nightshades - a category of foods which includes potatoes, tomatoes and tobacco

NMR - nuclear magnetic resonance (see MRI)

nociceptive - painful, injury producing

nucleus pulposis - the gelatin-like, water-binding center of an intervertebral disk

obliques - the two abdominal muscles which perform diagonal trunk flexion

occupational therapy - an allied medical profession concerned with functional activities for rehabilitation, developmental and psychiatric treatment

opposition - state in which body surfaces are in close proximity and parallel to each other, as with joint surfaces or thumb to finger pad

organic - physical; pertaining to the body

orthopedic - pertaining to the musculoskeletal system

orthopedic surgeon - an MD specializing in operations to correct conditions of the musculoskeletal system

orthopod - slang for orthopedic surgeon

osteoarthritis - condition characterized by localized degenerative changes in joints

osteophyte - bone spur

osteoporosis - abnormal thinning of the bones

osteopath - a graduate from a four-year school of osteopathic medicine with a DO degree

OT - occupational therapist or occupational therapy

pain behavior - actions and personality characteristics typical of patients whose chronic pain is reinforced by their environments

pain clinic - a rehabilitation center with a multidisciplinary approach to chronic pain

pain coping - therapeutic techniques to help chronic pain patients adjust to their disabilities

pain inhibition - techniques used to block the transmission of pain messages to the brain

pain management - therapeutic techniques to help chronic pain patients minimize their pain and maximize their function

palpation - examination by touch

paraspinal - in the area of the spine

paraspinal muscles - see spinal muscles

parasympathetic nervous system - the cranio-sacral portion of the autonomic nervous system

paravertebral - in the area of the vertebrae

paravertebral muscles - see spinal muscles

paresthesia - abnormal sensation, including pins-and-needles, tingling, burning

passive - performed by an outside force without active muscle contraction

pathology - diseased or abnormal state

pedicle - segment of the vertebral arch which joins the vertebral body to the lamina

pelvic obliquity - asymmetry of the pelvic ring creating a wind-blown effect

pelvic tilt - upward movement of the front of the pelvis which flattens the lumbar curve and which is accomplished by a contraction of the abdominal and gluteal muscles

pelvis - large bony ring joined to the spine at the sacrum and to the legs at the hip joints

perception - a person's knowledge of the physical world as interpreted by the brain

perianal - surrounding the anus

periosteum - outer covering of bone

peripheral - away from the central part of the body, usually referring to structures in the arms and legs

peripheral nervous system - the nerves of the body, peripheral to the spinal cord

perirectal - area surrounding the anus and end part of the rectum pharmacology - the study of drugs and their effects on the body

physiatrist - an MD specializing in physical medicine and non-surgical rehabilitation

physical therapy - an allied health profession which uses physical means to promote health and rehabilitation

pia mater - the innermost of the three meninges

piriformis - a muscle in the buttock through or under which the sciatic nerve passes

piriformis syndrome - a condition in which spasm of the piriformis muscle causes sciatic nerve compression

placebo - treatment which has no beneficial physical effects

placebo effect - relief of symptoms following the use of a placebo

posterior - toward the back of the body

posterior superior iliac spine - bony landmark on the pelvis near the top of the sacrum

posterolateral - angled toward the back and side of the body

post-op - following a surgical procedure

posture - the position one assumes against gravity

pre-op - preceding a surgical procedure

press-ups - an exercise of passive hyperextension in prone, used for disk prolapse

prognosis - outlook of an illness; chances for recovery

prolapsed disk - condition in which the nucleus of the disk pushes against the annular fibers, causing them to bulge into the spinal canal

proliferant - substance which stimulates the production of new tissue

prone - stomach-lying

protrusion - bulging of tissue beyond its normal boundary

PSIS - posterior superior iliac spine

psychiatrist - an MD specializing in treatment of emotional or mental problems

psychogenic - originating in the mind

PT - physical therapy or physical therapist

pubic symphysis - fibrous joint at the front of the pelvis

pubis - anterior part of the pelvis

pyriformis - see piriformis

Qi - Chinese concept meaning the body's vital energy

radiation - movement of symptoms from an injured area, often following the path of a nerve; electromagnetic waves

radicular - pertaining to a specific nerve root and its distribution

radiographic - pertaining to diagnostic tests in which x-rays or other electromagnetic waves are used to visualize internal parts of the body, including x-rays, CAT scans, MRI, myelograms, bone scans, etc.

radiologic/radiological - see radiographic

radiologist - an MD specializing in the performance and interpretation of radiographic testing

range of motion - the full arc of movement available at a joint

reciprocal inhibition - technique using a strong contraction of a tight muscle which causes subsequent inhibition and relaxation of that muscle

rectal tone - responsiveness of the sphincter muscles responsible for bowel retention

rectus - the abdominal muscle which performs straight trunk flexion

reflex - an immediate motor response following a sensory stimulus which initially bypasses the brain

reflex inhibition - reduction of muscle spasm through the use of nervous system mechanisms residency - hospital training for MDs or DOs following internship, for specialization

rheumatoid - pertaining to the joints of the body

ROM - see range of motion

rotation - twisting movement around a body axis

ruptured disk - a condition in which part of the nucleus of a disk has extruded through the outer annular fibers into the spinal canal

sacro-iliac joint - the connection between the pelvis and sacrum

sacro-iliac joint dysfunction - a syndrome in which the SI joint is subluxed, inflamed or painful

sacral - pertaining to the spinal region between the low back and tailbone

sacrum - five vertebrae located below the lumbar vertebrae which are fused into one bone

sciatica - pain which follows the path of the sciatic nerve down the back of the leg

sciatic nerve - large nerve composed of a bundle of nerve fibers from the lumbar and sacral parts of the spinal cord, which runs down the back of the thigh and innervates the posterior thigh, lower leg and foot

sclerotome - deep tissues which are innervated by the one spinal nerve

scoliosis - lateral curvature of the spine

secondary gains - benefits resulting from an illness

sensory stimulation - any input that sends messages about touch, temperature, vibration, movement, etc. through the sensory receptors to the central nervous system

sequestration - condition in which a fragment from the nucleus of a disk is loose in the spinal canal

sheath - outer covering of a nerve or muscle

SI - sacro-iliac

SIJ - sacro-iliac joint

SIJD - sacro-iliac joint dysfunction

SLR - straight leg raise

somatic - pertaining to the body

somatic dysfunction - term used in osteopathy to indicate a functional disorder of the musculoskeletal system

somatogenic - originating in the body

spasm - painful sustained contraction of a muscle in response to an injury to the muscle or to other nearby structures

specialist - an MD or DO who has completed a residency program in a specialty field

sphincter - muscle which allows retentive control of the bladder or bowel

spinal canal - the space within the vertebral column in which the spinal cord is located

spinal column - vertebral column; the bony spine

spinal cord - structure containing bundles of nerves which connects the brain and peripheral nervous system and which is enclosed by the spinal column

spinal muscles - four muscles composed of short fibers which originate and insert on the vertebrae and which extend and stabilize the spine

spinous process - posterior bony projection of a vertebra

spondylolysis - defect in the bony arch of a vertebra causing spinal instability

spondylolisthesis - bilateral defect of the bony arch of a vertebra with anterior slipping of the affected vertebral body

spondylosis - degenerative disease of the spine, with changes of vertebrae, joints and disks

sprain - injury or tearing of ligaments

stenosis - abnormal congenital or degenerative narrowing of the spinal canal

straight leg raise - a test for nerve root compression in which the hip is flexed with the knee extended; an exercise to stretch the hamstring muscle

straights - chiropractors who limit their practice to manipulation of the spinal column

strain - injury or tearing of muscle tissue

strain-counterstrain - a technique using passive positioning to reduce sensory input from soft tissues in order to reduce muscle tone

strength - the amount of resistance a muscle can overcome in a single repetition

structure - physical components of the body

subchondral bone - part of a bone located below the articular cartilage

subluxation - partial disruption of the opposing surfaces of a joint; slight vertebral malalignment

supine - back-lying

sympathetic nervous system - throacolumbar portion of the autonomic nervous system

symptom - a change in a patient's condition, indicating a dysfunctional state

syndrome - a set of symptoms which occur together, indicating a specific medical condition

synovial fluid - substance produced by the lining of a joint to provide shock-absorption, lubrication and protection for the joint

synovial joint - joint surrounded by a fluid-producing synovial membrane; a joint with a measurable amount of movement

synovial lining/membrane - the inner lining of a joint which secretes synovial fluid

systemic - affecting the whole body

tendon - non-elastic part of a muscle; inelastic cord which attaches a muscle to a bone

tendonitis - inflammation of a tendon

tenosynovitis - inflammation of a tendon and synovial membrane of a joint

TENS - see transcutaneous electrical nerve stimulation

therapeutic - beneficial; causing reversal of pathology or symptoms

thermograph - diagnostic tool which measures spinal heat

thoracic - pertaining to the trunk or to the part of the spine between the neck and waist

thrust - a sudden, high-velocity, low amplitude force applied to a specific structure of the body

tone - readiness of a muscle to contract; a muscle's resistance to stretch

total bedrest - see bedrest

toxic - poisonous to the body

traction - a pulling force which separates joint surfaces

transcutaneous electrical nerve stimulation - a modality which imparts a mild electrical current to the skin to inhibit pain elsewhere in the body

transverse ligaments - short ligaments connecting the transverse processes of two vertebrae

transverse process - bony lateral projection of a vertebra to which muscles and ligaments attach

trigger point - most tender spot in a muscle; tender area of fibrous bands in a muscle

trochanter - bony prominence on the femur

trochanteric belt - stabilizing support which surrounds the pelvis at hip level to provide support for the SI joint

tropism - degenerative scoliosis of individual spinal segments caused by asymmetry of disks or vertebrae

ultra-sound - machine which uses sound waves to produce heat in deep tissues

Valsalva maneuver - tightening of the abdominal muscles with a closed glottis; straining

vascular - having a large blood supply

vertebra - single bony segment of the spinal column

vertebrae - plural of vertebra

vertebral body - the largest part of a vertebra, separated from other vertebral bodies by disks
vertebral column - spinal column; bony spine
vertebral process - one of a number of bony projections of a vertebra
viscera - the large interior organs of the body

Williams flexion exercises - treatment regime for low back pain which emphasizes flexion postures and abdominal strengthening
work hardening - a treatment program which simulates a patient's work environment in order to return injured workers to the job safely and quickly

x-ray - a radiographic test in which the bones of the body are visualized

yin and yang - names for the Chinese concept of the two opposing influences on the body

Appendix B

Bibliography

Abraham, Edward, *Freedom from Back Pain: An Orthopedist's Self-Help Guide*, Rodale, 1986

Allen, Henry, "That Back's Gotta Come Out," *The Washington Post,* April 29, 1990

American Medical Association, *The American Medical Association Book of Back Care*, Random House, 1982

American Osteopathic Association, informational literature, 1987-1989

"Approaches to Musculoskeletal Problems: Focus on the Low Back," Robert M. True, M.D. Symposium, April 26-27, 1985, South Portland, Maine

Apts, David & Blankenship, Keith, *Back Facts for the American Back School*, FPR, Inc., 1981

The Back Letter, "Memo on Body Mechanics," Ed. Theresa Reger, Skol Publishing

The Back Letter, Ed. Theresa Reger, Skol Publishing, Vol. 4, No. 2-9, December 1989-July, 1990

Barnes, John, "Benefits of Myofascial Release, Craniosacral Therapy Explained," *Physical Therapy Forum*, Aug., 29, 1984

Barnes, John, "Pro: Never Trademarked Myofascial Release," *P.T. Bulletin*, Feb. 17, 1988

Barnes, John, "Therapeutic Insight," *Physical Therapy Forum*, June 25, 1986

Batson, Glenna, "Reeducating or Strengthening: Relooking at the Pelvic Tilt," *Physical Therapy Forum*, Oct. 2, 1985

Beal, Myron, "The Sacroiliac Problem: Review of Anatomy, Mechanics and Diagnosis," *Journal of Amer. Osteopathic Assoc.*, Vol. 81, No. 10, June, 1982

Bellamy, Nicholas, Park, William & Rooney, Patrick, "What Do We Know About the Sacroiliac Joint," *Seminars in Arthritis and Rheumatism*, Vol. 12, No. 3, February, 1983

Benanti, Joseph & Ellis, Jeffrey, "Holistic Medicine a 'Crisis' for PTs," *PT Bulletin*, Jan. 18, 1989

Benjamin, Ben, "The Mystery of Lower Back Pain," Parts I & II, *Massage Therapy Journal*, Fall 1988 & Winter 1989

Blackburn, Stan & Portney, Leslie Gross, "Electromyographic Activity of Back Musculature During Williams' Flexion Exercises," Physical Therapy, Vol. 61, No. 6, June, 1981

Brena, Steven F., *Chronic Pain: America's Hidden Epidemic*, Atheneum/SMI, 1978

Bunch, Richard, "Con: Myofascial Release Traced Back Decades," *P.T. Bulletin*, Feb. 17, 1988

Burkart, Sandy & Beresford, William, "The Aging Intervertebral Disk," *Physical Therapy*, Vol. 59, No. 8, August, 1979

Cailliet, Rene, *Low Back Pain Syndrome*, Second Edition, F.A. Davis, 1962

Cailliet, Rene, *Low Back Pain Syndrome*, Edition 4, F.A. Davis, 1988

Caplan, Deborah, *Back Trouble*, Triad Publishing Co., 1987

Carmichael, Joel, "Inter- and Intra-Examiner Reliability of Palpation for Sacroiliac Joint Dysfunction," *Journal of Manipulative and Physiological Therapeutics*, Vol. 10, No. 4, August, 1987

Carper, Jean, *Health Care U.S.A.*, Prentice Hall Press, 1987

Carr, Sharon & Phillips, Cathy L.,"Helping TMJ Patients to Help Themselves," *Physical Therapy Forum*, Jan. 8, 1990

Carroll, Sarah, "Hypnosis: An Underutilized Modality," *Physical Therapy Forum*

Carter, Mildred, *Helping Yourself With Foot Reflexology*, Parker Publishing Co., 1969

Cassel, Eric, "The Nature of Suffering and the Goals of Medicine," *New England Journal of Medicine*, Vol. 306, No. 11, March 18, 1982

Chapman-Smith, David, "Chiropractic – A Referenced Source of Modern Concepts, New Evidence," Practice Makers Products Inc., 1988

CIBA Clinical Symposia,"Low Back Pain," Vol. 25, Number 3, CIBA Pharmaceutical Co., 1973

Cibulka, Michael & Koldehoff, Rhonda, "Evaluating Chronic Sacroiliac Joint Dysfunction," *Clinical Management*, Vol. 6, No. 4, 1987

Cibulka, Michael & Koldehoff, Rhonda, "Leg Length Disparity and Its Effect on Sacroiliac Joint Dysfunction," *Clinical Management*, Vol. 6, No. 5, 1987

Colbin, Annemarie, *Food and Healing*, Ballantine Books, 1986

Consumer Reports Books, Editors of, *Health Quackery: Consumers Union's Report on False Health Claims, Worthless Remedies and Unproved Therapies*, Holt, Rhinehart and Winston, 1980

Cousins, Norman, *Anatomy of an Illness*, W.W. Norton & Co., 1979

Croce, Pat, "Put Stress to Rest," *Physical Therapy Forum*, August 21, 1989

Cuckler, John, Bernini, Philip, Wiesel, Sam, Booth, Robert, Ruthman, Richard & Pickens, Gary, "The Use of Epidural Steroids in the Treatment of Lumbar Radicular Pain," *The Journal of Bone & Joint Surgery*, Vol. 67-A, No. 1, January, 1985

Cyriax, James, *Textbook of Orthopaedic Medicine*, Baillier-Tindall, 1980

Derebery, Jane & Tullis, William, "Delayed Recovery in the Patient with a Work Compensable Injury," *Journal of Occupational Medicine*, Nov., 1983

Deyo, Richard, "Conservative Therapy for Low Back Pain," *JAMA*, Aug. 26, 1983, Vol. 250

Deyo, Richard, Loeser, John & Bigos, Stanley, "Herniated Lumbar Intervertebral Disk," *Annals of Internal Medicine*, Vol. 112, No. 8, April 15, 1990

Deyo, Richard, Walsh, Nicholas, Martin, Donald, Schoenfeld, Lawrence & Ramamurthy, Somayaji, "A Controlled Trial of Transcutaneous Electrical Nerve Stimulation (TENS) and Exercise for Chronic Low Back Pain," *The New England Journal of Medicine*, Vol. 322, No. 23, June 7, 1990

DiFabio, Richard, "Clinical Assessment of Manipulation and Mobilization of the Lumbar Spine," *Physical Therapy*, Vol. 66, No. 1, Jan., 1986

Dimick, Terry, "Kinesiotherapist Responds," *P.T. Bulletin*, July 4, 1990

Dommerholt, Jan, "Meridian Therapy – A New European Concept," *Physical Therapy Forum*, March 5, 1990

DonTigny, Richard, "Dysfunction of the Sacroiliac Joint and Its Treatment," *The Journal of Orthopaedic and Sports Medicine Therapy*, Vol. 1, No. 1, Summer, 1979

DonTingy, Richard, "Function and Pathomechanics of the Sacroiliac Joint," *Physical Therapy*, Vol. 65, No. 1, Jan., 1985

Edgelow, Peter, "Physical Examination of the Lumbosacral Complex," *Physical Therapy*, Vol. 59, No. 8, Aug., 1979

Elgee, Neil, "Norman Cousins' Sick Laughter Redux," *Archives of Internal Medicine*, Vol. 150, August, 1990

Fager, Charles, "Beware the Quick Fix for Back Pain," *Trends in Rehabilitation*, Winter, 1986

Fager, Charles, "Facts and Fallacies of Spinal Disorders: A Neurosurgeon's Viewpoint," *Evaluation and Treatment of Chronic Pain*

Fager, Charles, "The Neurosurgical Management of Lumbar Spine Disease," *New Developments in Medicine*, Vol. 3, No. 2, Sept., 1988

Fahey, Brian, "The Principles of Structural Diagnosis," *Physical Therapy Forum*, Oct. 23, 1989

Folan, Lilias, *Lilias Yoga and You*, Bantum Books, 1972

Friedman, Nancy, "Back Exercises for a Healthy Back," Krames Communications, 1985

Gildenberg, Philip L. & DeVaul, Richard A., *The Chronic Pain Patient*, Kargen, 1985

Glade, Phyllis, *Crystal Healing: The Next Step*, Llewellyn Publications, 1989

Glisan, Billy, Stith, William & Kiser, Sanford, "Physiology of Active Exercise in Rehabilitation of Back Injuries," *Health Tracks*, Vol. 2, Issue 1

Goering, Gail, "Treat Injured Workers Like Athletes," *P.T. Bulletin*, May 9, 1990

Gottlieb, Harold, Alperson, Burton, Koller, Reuben & Hockersmith, Virgil, "An Innovative Program for the Restoration of Patients with Chronic Back Pain," *Physical Therapy*, Vol. 59, No. 8, August, 1979

Grieve, Elizabeth "Lumbo-pelvic Rhythm and Mechanical Dysfunction of the Sacro-iliac Joint," *Physiotherapy*, Vol. 67, No. 6, June, 1981

Hay, Louise, *You Can Heal Your Life*, Hay House, 1984

Headley, Barbara, *Chronic Pain: Life Out of Balance*, H. Duane Saunders, 1987

Headley, Barbara, "Dynamic Stabilization," *Physical Therapy Forum*, June 4, 1990

Headley, Barbara, "Pain Vs. Suffering," *Physical Therapy Forum*, May 16, 1988

Headley, Barbara, "Postural Homeostasis," *Physical Therapy Forum*, Sept. 17, 1990

Hebert, Lauren, *Sex and Back Pain*, H. Duane Saunders, 1987

Heinrich, Steve, "Body Watch: The Importance of Dialogue and Myofascial Unwinding in Creating a Safe Place to Heal," *Physical Therapy Forum*, Feb. 5, 1990

Heller, Joseph & Hanson, Jan, *The Client's Handbook*, The Body of Knowledge, Mt. Shasta, Ca.

Horwich, Mark, "Low Back Pain: The Neurologist's View," *Drug Therapy*, Dec., 1982

Hutchinson, Lynn, "Direct Access and Preventative Therapy," *Physical Therapy Forum*, Sept., 25, 1989

Imrie, David, *Goodbye Back Ache*, Prentice-Hall/Newcastle, 1983

Irwin, Yukiko, *Shiatzu*, J.B. Lippincott, 1976

Ishmael, William & Shorbe, Howard, "Care of the Back," J.B. Lippincott Co., 1953

Jackson, Claudia & Brown, Mark, "Analysis of Current Approaches and a Practical Guide to Prescription of Exercise," *Clinical Orthopaedics*, No. 179, October, 1983

Jackson, Claudia & Brown, Mark, "Is There a Role for Exercise in the Treatments of Patients with Low Back Pain," *Clinical Orthopaedics*, No. 179, October, 1983

Jacobs, Bernard, "Low Back Pain: The Orthopedist's View," *Drug Therapy*, Dec., 1982

Jones, Bob, *The Difference a D.O. Makes*, Osteopathic Medicine in the Twentieth Century, Times-Journal Publishing Co., Oklahoma City, Ok., 1978

Jones, Frank Pierce, *Body Awareness in Action: A Study of the Alexander Technique*, Schocken Books, 1979

Kaplan, Paul & Tanner, Ellen, *Musculoskeletal Pain and Disability*, Appleton & Lange, 1989

Kessler, Randolph, "Acute Symptomatic Disk Prolapse," *Physical Therapy*, Vol. 59, No. 8, Aug., 1979

Kessler, Randolph & Hertling, Darlene, *Management of Common Musculoskeletal Disorders*,

Harper & Row, 1983

Kim, Nini, "Holistic Medicine Requires Different World View," *PT Bulletin*, March 1, 1989

Kirkaldy-Willis, W.H., *Managing Low Back Pain*, Churchill Livingstone, 1988

Kirkaldy-Willis, W.H. & Hill, R.J., "A More Precise Diagnosis for Low Back Pain," *Spine*, Vol. 4, No. 2, Mar./Apr., 1979

Klein, Arthur & Sobel, Dava, *Backache Relief*, New American Library, 1985

Knott, Margaret & Voss, Dorothy, *Proprioceptive Neuramuscular Facilitation*, Harper & Row, 1968

Kotzsch, Ronald, "AIDS: Putting an Alternative to the Test," *East West*, Sept., 1986

Krumhansl, Bernice & Nowacek, Charles, "Case Study – Spinal Manipulation Under Anaesthesia," *Physical Therapy Forum*, Sept. 4, 1989

Lamb, David, "The Neurology of Spinal Pain," *Physical Therapy*, Vol. 59, No. 8, Aug., 1979

Langone, John, *Chiropractors: A Consumer's Guide*, Addison-Wesley Publishing Co., 1982

Lauterback, Joyce, "The Mind-Body Connection – Is There More?" *Physical Therapy Forum*, July 17, 1989

Lawn, George, "How to Lift – Is There a Right Way?" *Physical Therapy Forum*, June 12, 1985

Lehman, Betsy, "Feeling Bad About Feeling Bad," *The Good Health Magazine (Boston Globe)*, October 8, 1989

Levine, David B., *The Painful Low Back*, Merck, Sharp & Dohme, 1979

Lewith, Geroge & Horn, Sandra, *Drug Free Pain Relief*, Thorsons Publishers, 1987

Lockett, Ricky, "Pyriformis Syndrome – Diagnosis and Treatment," *Physical Therapy Forum*, Aug. 22, 1988

MacPhee, Patricia, "Chronic Pain and the Role of Occupational Therapy," *Physical Therapy Forum*, Sept. 18, 1989

Maitland, G.D., *Vertebral Manipulation*, Butterworths, 1977

Marantz, Steve, "The Perfect Chair," *The Boston Globe*, Oct. 8, 1989

Mayer, Tom, "Rehabilitation of the Patient with Spinal Pain," *The Orthopedic Clinics of North America*, Vol. 14, No. 3, July 1983

McGavin, James, "The McKenzie Approach to Spinal Pain," *Physical Therapy Forum*, July 5, 1988

McKenzie, Robin, *Treat Your Own Back*, Spinal Publications Ltd., 1985

McGregor, Marion & Cassidy, David, "Post-surgical Sacroiliac Joint Syndrome," *Journal of Manipulative and Physiologic Therapeutics*, Vol. 6, No. 1, March, 1983

Mead, Mark, "Chiropractic's New Wave," *East West*, November, 1989

Melnick, Michael, Saunders, Robin & Saunders, Duane, *Managing Back Pain*, H. Duane Saunders, 1989

Miller, David, "Comparison of Electromyographic Activity in the Lumbar Paraspinal Muscles of Subjects with and without Low Back Pain," *Physical Therapy*, Vol. 65, No. 9, Sept., 1985

Mills, Simon & Finando, Steven, *Alternatives in Healing: An Open-Minded Approach to Finding the Best Treatment for Your Health Problems*, New American Library, 1989

Mixter, Jason, "Rolfing," (Editors) Lowe & Nechas, *Whole Body Healing*, Rodale Press, 1983

Montgomery, Edith, "Folsom Physical Therapy – A Different Approach to Back Rehabilitation," *Physical Therapy Forum*, June 13, 1988

Olsen, Paulette, "Body Mechanics Education – A Legacy for our Children," *Physical Therapy Forum*, April 23, 1990

Olsen, Paulette, "Brief Media Presentations on Back Care," *Physical Therapy Forum*, Nov. 27, 1989

Ondricek, Jana, "Techniques for Effective Therapeutic Management of Workmen's Compensation Patients," *Physical Therapy Forum*, April 30, 1990

Ongley, Milne, Klein, Robert, Dorman, Thomas, Eek, Bjorn, & Hubert, Lawrence, "A New Approach to the Treatment of Chronic Back Pain," *The Lancet*, July 18, 1987

Paris, Stanley, "Anatomy as Related to Function and Pain," *The Orthopedic Clinics of North America*, Vol. 14, No. 3, July, 1983

Paris, Stanley, "Mobilization of the Spine," *Physical Therapy*, Vol. 59, No. 8, Aug., 1979

Paris, Stanley, "Physical Signs of Instability," *Spine*, Vol. 10, No. 3, 1985

Paris, Stanley, *The Spine*, (Course Notes), Stanley Paris, 1979

Picker, Robert, "Microcurrent Therapy: 'Jump-Starting' Healing with Bioelectricity," *Physical Therapy Forum*, June 10, 1989

Pitzele, Sefra Korbin, *We Are Not Alone: Learning to Live with Chronic Illness*, Workman Publishing, 1985

Potter, Nancy & Rothstein, Jules, "Intertester Reliability for Selected Clinical Tests of the Sacroiliac Joint," *Physical Therapy*, Vol. 65, No. 11, Nov., 1985

Prudden, Bonnie, *Pain Erasure*, Ballantine Books, 1980

P.T. Bulletin, "Benefits of 'Humor Therapy' Promoted," April 25, 1980

P.T. Bulletin, "Reactions Mixed to Back Surgery Alternative," August 30, 1989

Rashbaum, Ralph, "Radiofrequency Facet Denervation," *The Orthopedic Clinics of North America*, Vol. 14, No. 3, July, 1983

Reese, David, "Keep PT the Art That It Is," *P.T. Bulletin*, April 25, 1990

Register, Cheri, *Living with Chronic Illness: Days of Patience and Passion*, The Free Press (Maacmillan), 1987

Reuben, Carolyn, "AIDS: The Promise of Alternative Treatments," *East West*, Sept., 1986

Rice, John, Allen, Nancy & Caldwell, David, "Low Back Pain: The Rheumatologist's View," *Drug Therapy*, Dec., 1982

Richardson, Nancy, "Aston-Patterning," *Physical Therapy Forum*, Oct., 28, 1987

Rolf, Ida, "Structural Integration," *Confin. Psychiat.* 16, 1973

Sarno, John, *Mind Over Back Pain*, Berkley Books, 1982

Saunders, H. Duane, *The Back Care Program*, H. Duane Saunders, 1983

Saunders, H. Duane, *Evaluation, Treatment and Prevention of Musculoskeletal Disorders*, H. Duane Saunders, 1985

Saunders, Duane, *For Your Neck*, H. Duane Saunders, 1986

Shapiro, Gary, "Ceasing the Struggle," *Physical Therapy Forum*, May 7, 1990

Shea, Michael, "MFR and the Psychosomatic Body," *Physical Therapy Forum*, April 23, 1990

Sherman, Carl, "The Medicolegal Thicket of Low Back Disability," *Aches and Pains*, April, 1982

Siegel, Bernie S., *Peace, Love and Healing*, Harper & Row, 1989

Simons, David & Travell, Janet, "Myofascial Origins of Low Back Pain," Parts 1-3, *Postgraduate Medicine*, Vol. 73, No. 2, Feb., 1983

Smith, Ralph Lee, *At Your Own Risk: The Case Against Chiropractic*, Trident Press, 1969

Solet, Jo, "Low Back Pain – An Overview," *Physical Therapy Forum*, August 7, 1989

Steer, Allen, Hardin, John & Malawista, Stephen, "Lyme Arthritis: A New Clinical Entity," *Hospital Practice*, April, 1978

Sternbach, Richard A., *Pain Patients; Traits and Treatments*, Academic Press, 1974

Stickland, Ellen, "Trouble with KTs," *PT Bulletin*

Tamayo, Rey, "Work Hardening – A Different Treatment Approach," *Physical Therapy Forum*, Feb. 26, 1990

Thomas, Lynn, Hislop, Helen & Waters, Robert, "Physiological Work Performance in Chronic Low Back Disability," *Physical Therapy*, Vol. 60, No. 4, April, 1980

Wallnofer, Heinrich & vonRottauscher, Anna, *Chinese Folk Medicine and Acupuncture*, Bell Publishing Co., 1965

Weiselfish, Sharon & Kain, Jay, "Introduction of Developmental Manual Therapy – An Integrated System Approach for Structural and Functional Rehabilitation," *Physical Therapy Forum*, Feb. 12, 1990

White, Arthur, "Injection Techniques for the Diagnosis and Treatment of Low Back Pain," *The Orthopedic Clinics of North America*, Vol. 14, No. 3, July, 1983

Wildman, Frank, "The Feldenkrais Method: Clinical Applications," *P.T. Forum*, Feb. 19, 1986

Wildman, Frank, "Learning – The Missing Link in Physical Therapy," *P.T. Forum*, Feb. 8, 1988

Wildman, Frank, "Training in the Feldenkrais Method," The Institute for Movement Studies, Berkeley, Ca.

Wilk, Chester, *Chiropractic Speaks Out*, Wilk Publishing Co., 1973

Willis, Judith, "Back Pain: Ubiquitous, Controversial," *FDA Consumer*, November, 1983

Wolf, Barbara, *Living With Pain*, The Seabury Press, 1977

Woodworth, Barbara, "Therapeutic Values of Tai Chi," *Physical Therapy Forum*, July 23, 1990

Wyatt, William, DO, literature for patients, 1987

Yunus, Muhammed, Masi, Alfonse, Calabro, John & Shah, Indravadan, "Primary Fibromyalgia," *Amer. Fam. Phys.*, May, 1982

Zacharkow, Dennis, "The Problems with Lumbar Support," *Physical Therapy Forum*, Sept. 10, 1990

Zimmerman, Julie, *Goals and Objectives for Developing Normal Movement Patterns*, Aspen, 1988

Zinman, David, "Focus on Back Pain," *Newsday*, Jan. 30, 1990

Index - The Almanac of Back Pain Treatments

drugs (see addiction, medications)
dysfunction 35-6, 38, 40; diagnosis of d. 36; somatic d. 38-9; treatment 113
dura 120

electrotherapy 53-4, 68
emotional/psychological factors, e./p. effects of pain 107, 109; e./p. effects on recovery 140, 145-50; e./p. effects of treatment 52-3; e./p. f.s contributing to pain 146, 148-9; treatment 109-10, 121-2, 146-50
endorphins 8, 25, 102, 114, 147, 149
endurance 88, 101
energy flow 47-8, 121, 140, 148
epidural injection (see injection)
equipment, exercise 57-8; positioning e. 57-8; seating e. 57, 80-1 [Fig. 8-2]; (see biofeedback; electrotherapy)
erector spinae 90-3, 96-7 [Fig. 9-1]
ergonomics 106
exercise (see physical conditioning)
exercises for disk prolapse 96-7 [Fig. 9-3]; for endurance 88; extension e.s 96-7; for flexibility 87-8, 96, 102; flexion e.s. 36, 90, 93-6 [Fig. 9-2]; guidelines 87-9; individualization of e.s 36, 87, 90, 99, 154; neck e.s 97; in movement patterns 99; positioning for e.s 89; for strengthening 88-9
extension 91, 96 (see exercises, extension)

facet joints 15, 21-2, 90, 96, 116 [Fig. 1-6, 1-7, 1-8 C]; f. j. dysfunction 25, 29-30 [Fig. 1-11]; treatment 68-9, 111-3
family doctor 33-5
fascia 21, 29, 48, 119-23, 126
fat (see diet)
feelings (see attitude; emotional/psych. factors)
Feldenkrais 126-7
financial cost of back pain 6 (see workers' compensation)
fitness programs 102-4 (see physical conditioning)
flexibility (see exercises, flex.; range of motion)
flexion 22, 90-1 (see exercises, flexion)
foot reflexology 136
friction massage (see massage)
functional mobility 115-6
functional restoration (see work hardening)
fusion, spinal 66

gate control theory 23, 133
gluteals 91-3. 97 [Fig. 9-1]
gravity, effects on body 77, 125-6; effects on exercise 89

hamstrings 91-4, 97 [Fig. 9-1]
Hay, Louise 148
heat 53, 155
Hellerwork 128-9
herbalism 141-2

hip joint [Fig. 1-2]; muscles of h. j. 91, 97 [Fig. 9-1]
holism 47-8, 62
homeopathy 141-2
humor 147, 150, 155
hypnosis 72, 149

ice 53-4, 155
ilium (pl. ilia) 15 [Fig. 1-2]
individualization of treatment 9, 36, 46-8, 87, 90, 99, 104, 110, 153-4, 156-7
inflammation 29; treatment 52-4, 61-2, 155
inhibition (see muscle i.; pain i.)
injections 68-9
instability (see facet joint dysfunction, sacro-iliac joint dysfunc.)
internship 33
intervertebral disks (see disks)
intra-abdominal pressure 93
ischium 15 [Fig. 1-2]
isometrics 89, 93, 97

job injuries (see work injuries; workers' compensation)
jogging 103
joint capsule 15 [Fig. 1-8]; pinching of 113
joint dysfunction (see facet jnt. dysf., SIJ dysf.)
joint play 22, 113
joints 15, 21-2 [Fig. 1-8]

kinesiologists/kinesiology 154
kinesiotherapists/therapy 36-7
kyphosis 13

laughter (see humor)
Law of the Nerve 40-1
lifestyle changes 52, 79-80, 140, 156
lifting 81-4 [Fig. 8-3, 8-4]
ligaments 15, 77, 79; sprain 29, 77, 79, 115; (see soft tissues)
locked back (see facet joint dysfunction)
longitudinal ligaments 15 [Fig. 1-4, 1-7]
lordosis 13, 80, 93-4 [Fig. 8-1, 8-2]
low back syndrome 6, 10, 25, 34
lumbar roll 80-1 [Fig. 8-2]
lumbar spine 13 [Fig. 1-1]; l. support [Fig. 8-2]; (see lordosis)
lying down 82

macrobiotics 140
magnetic resonance imaging 65-6
malalignment (see asymmetry; dysfunction; subluxation)
manipulation 111-8, 155; chiropractic m. 39-43, 46, 112, 121; m. under anesthesia 69; osteopathic m. 37-9, 46, 112, 120
manual therapy (see manipulation; mobilization)

179

pain 21-5; p. clinics 36, 107-10; p. coping/management 36, 107-10; p. inhibition 54, 61, 68, 102, 114, 132-3; (see chronic p.; perception)
pain-killers (see injections; medications)
pelvic tilts 80, 90, 93
pelvis 15 [Fig. 1-2]
perception of pain 21-5, 107-9
personality and pain (see attitude; emotional/psych. factors)
physiatrists 34, 36, 46, 154
physical conditioning 79, 101-4, 155
physical fitness instructors 103-4
physical therapists/therapy 35-6, 46, 122-3, 154
physicians (see medical doctors; osteopathic doctors)
piriformis muscle 29-30 [Fig. 1-13]
piriformis syndrome 29
placebo effect 8, 24-5, 117, 146, 149
positioning 80, 155; equipment for p. 57-8 [Fig. 8-2]; in bed 53, 82; in lifting 81-2 [Fig. 8-3, 8-4]; in sitting 57-8, 80-1, 84 [Fig. 8-2]; in standing 81 [Fig. 8-1]
positive attitude (see attitude)
posterior longitudinal ligaments (see longitudinal lig.s)
posture/body mechanics 51, 57, 77-85, 99, 102, 127-8, 155 [Fig. 8-1, 8-2, 8-3, 8-4]
press-ups 97 [Fig. 9-3]
prevalence of back pain 6
prevention of back pain 38, 42, 79, 101
prolapse, disk (see disks)
proprioceptive neuromuscular facilitation 129
psychiatrists/psychiatry 34 (see counseling)
psychological (see emotional/psych. factors)
psychotherapy (see counseling)
public symphysis 15 [Fig. 1-2]
pubis 15 [Fig. 1-2]

radiation of symptoms 30, 66
radiofrequency facet denervation 68
radiographic tests 65-6 [Fig. 6-2]
radiologic tests (see radiographic tests)
range of motion 21-2, 73-4, 79, 87-8
referral of patients 33-6, 46-7, 157
reflexes 21
reflex inhibition 73, 114
reflexology (see foot reflexology)
rehabilitation following work injury 105-7
relaxants, muscle (see medications)
relaxation techniques 71-5, 149, 155
residency 33
resistance exercises 89
responsibility of patient 9-10, 47, 80, 106-10, 145-50, 154-6, 158
rest 82 (see balance of rest/activity; bedrest)
rheumatologists 34
rhizotomy 68

Structural Integration (see Rolfing)
subluxation 40-2, 46, 116, 121 (see facet joint dysfunction)
suction for disk removal 67
supports (see equipment, seating)
surgery 65-9, 155
survey of back pain people 45-6, 104
swimming 102-3
symptomatic treatment 34 (see pain inhibition)
synovial joints 15, 21-2 [Fig. 1-8 C]
synovial membrane 15 [Fig. 1-8 C]

Tai Chi 73
tendons 21, 29, 75 [Fig. 1-8]
TENS (see transcutaneous electrical nerve stimulation)
tension, emotional/muscular 46, 107, 120-1, 126, 146, 155; treatment 61-2, 71-3, 102, 108-10, 121-2, 126-9, 146, 155
tension myositis syndrome 146
therapy (see physical t.; occupational t.; kinesiot.)
thermography 40
thoracic spine 13 [Fig. 1-1]; t. support [Fig. 8-2]
thrust (see manipulation)
TMS (see tension myositis syndrome)
traction 54-5, 133-4
Trager therapy 129
tranquilizers (see medications)
transcutaneous electrical nerve stimulation 54
treatment, goals of 9-10, 153-4, 157
trigger points 134-6

ultrasound (see heat)
unwinding (see somatoemotional release)

Valium (see medications)
vertebra (pl. -ae) 13-5, 29 [Fig. 1-1, 1-3, 1-4, 1-5, 1-6, 1-7, 1-9]
vertebral bodies 15 [Fig. 1-4, 1-5, 1-6, 1-7]
vertebral column (see spinal column)
Veterans hospitals 36-7
visualization 72, 149
vitamin therapy 139, 141
vocational rehab 108 (see work hardening)

walking 102-3
weakness (see muscle w.)
weight loss 52, 80
Williams flexion exercises (see exercises, flexion)
work injuries 36, 52, 105-7, 155
work hardening 36, 105-7, 155
workers' compensation 6

x-rays 34, 40-2, 66, 115-6

The Diagnosis and Misdiagnosis of Back Pain

A complete guide to the causes of bad backs and how professionals
diagnose them, by Julie Zimmerman, PT.

Table of Contents

Chronic Back Pain: Moving On

A complete guide to the treatment and management options for people living with bad backs, by Julie Zimmerman, PT.

Table of Contents

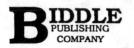

Order Form

Please send

_____ copies of *The Diagnosis and Misdiagnosis of
Back Pain* at $9.95 each $ _____

_____ copies of *The Almanac of Back Pain Treatments*
at $9.95 each $ _____

_____ copies of *Chronic Back Pain: Moving On*
at $9.95 each $ _____

                                            Subtotal $ _____

For orders of 3-5 books, deduct 15%
For orders of 6 or more books, deduct 20%.   – _____

Sales in state of Maine, add 5% sales tax.   + _____

Shipping, add $1.75 for first book, and $.75 for
each additional book.   + _____

                                    Total enclosed $ _____

Send check payable to: Biddle Publishing Company
                        Box 1305 - #103
                        Brunswick, Maine 04011

Expect up to four weeks for delivery.

For inquiries regarding discounts on larger orders, call 207-833-5016.